Toxic Substances and Mental Retardation

Monographs of the American Association on Mental Deficiency, 8

Michael J. Begab, Series Editor

Toxic Substances and Mental Retardation

Neurobehavioral Toxicology and Teratology

Edited by

Stephen R. Schroeder
University of North Carolina

Published by
American Association on Mental Deficiency
1719 Kalorama Road, NW
Washington, DC 20009

No. 8, Monographs of the American Association on Mental Deficiency (ISSN 0098-7123)

Library of Congress Cataloging-in-Publication Data

Toxic substances and mental retardation.

(Monographs of the American Association of Mental Deficiency, ISSN 0098-7123; 8)
Includes bibliographies.
1. Mental retardation—Etiology. 2. Behavioral toxicology. 3. Neurotoxic agents. 4. Fetal alcohol syndrome—Complications and sequelae. 5. Lead-poisoning—Complications and sequelae. I. Schroeder, Stephen R. II. Series: Monographs of the American Association on Mental Deficiency; no. 8. [DNLM: 1. Abnormalities, Drug Induced. 2. Behavior—drug effects. 3. Mental Retardation—etiology. 4. Teratogens. W1 MO569QMC no. 8/WM 300 T755]

RC570.T68 1987 616.85′88071 87-1776
ISBN 0-940898-15-2 (pbk.)

Printed in the United States of America

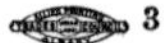 3

Dedication

This volume is dedicated to my wife, Carolyn, my favorite spouse, colleague, and sometimes-teacher.

Table of Contents

Foreword

Toxic substances loom large on the horizon as threats to the preservation of life on our planet. Of paramount concern are those toxins that attack the central nervous system causing death, encephalopathy, or mental retardation. The range and prevalence of toxicants is growing at an exponential rate, not only among the industrialized, but also the nonindustrialized third-world countries. The fields of neurobehavioral toxicology and teratology have been largely the province of the public health and occupational medicine professions. They have received little attention from the field of mental retardation. Mental retardation professionals must get involved *now* or abdicate their role in shaping public policy on the use of toxic substances to make it consistent with contemporary views of mental retardation.

The present monograph attempts to bring together disparate lines of research, theory, and practice from the areas of neurobehavioral toxicology and teratology in order to make practitioners in mental retardation aware of relevant theories and methodologies and in order to make researchers in mental retardation aware of the clinical sequelae of neurotoxicity. Researchers active in the field were invited to contribute not encyclopedic reviews of their subspecialties, but rather descriptions of their own work as examples of the appropriate methodologies for framing the questions and interpreting results correctly.

One of the hallmarks of neurotoxicity is the ubiquity of its expression. Multiple organ systems are often affected. Patients often suffer from neurotoxic effects before overt symptoms can be observed. Each toxicant also has it own peculiar effects that require multimodal methods of assessment to detect.

The first two chapters primarily discuss toxic effects on the fetus. Streissguth and LaDue explore the differential diagnosis of Fetal Alcohol Syndrome. Of particular interest is their description of a continuum of effects characterized by growth deficiency, dysmorphism, and central nervous system aberrations. Gualtieri's chapter uses quite a different methodology, retrospective analyses of very large databases, to make inferences about immunoreactivity theory. His basic conclusion is that fetal immune protection is relative, not absolute. It stongly suggests that assessments of pre- and perinatal complications take into account the sex of the proband, antecedent siblings, and the family proclivity to autoimmune and to allergic disorders.

The next three chapters are concerned with lead effects on infancy and childhood. Lead research has often been the proving ground for future studies of neurotoxicity in other areas, such as polychlorinated biphenyls, methyl mercury, cadmium, and multiple exposures to toxic waste. The first chapter of this set, by Dietrich, Krafft, Shukla, Bornschein, and Succop, is a good prototype of the ten prospective longitudinal studies of early lead exposure currently being conducted around the world. It also presents an excellent example of the care needed in selecting a proper sample, adequately documenting exposure history, and performing the necessary complex statistical procedures required for analysis of such longitudinal studies. The Schroeder and Hawk chapter takes a cross-sectional approach that explores the relationships between the neurotoxic effects of lead exposure and the many confounding social factors that occur as covariates of lead. The Otto chapter explores various electrophysiological measures that show promise as culture-free measures of neurotoxicity. Considerable work remains to be done, in order to relate these findings to the clinical behavioral phenomena.

The Guthrie and Young chapter discusses various prevention methodologies, goals for prevention, cost-benefit analyses, and a concrete model of a state plan for prevention.

Clearly, the key to coping with the effects of all of the toxic substances treated in this volume is prevention. The hazards they create will not await our development of an elegant research paradigm or intervention plan. They are happening *now*. As Leon Eisenberg (1977) has put it, "Not to act is to act."

REFERENCES

Eisenberg, L. (1977). The social imperatives of medical research. *Science, 198,* 1105–1110.

Quotation

Crafty men condemn studies; simple men admire them; and wise men use them; for they teach not their own use; but that is a wisdom without them, and above them, won by observation. Read not to contradict and confute; nor to believe and take for granted; nor to find talk and discourse; but to weigh and consider.

Francis Bacon

Fetal Alcohol

Teratogenic Causes of Developmental Disabilities

Ann P. Streissguth
and
Robin A. LaDue

University of Washington
School of Medicine

Most causes of mental retardation and developmental disability are unknown. In such cases, we are left with the task of describing and providing recommendations for disabilities that are diverse in cause, varied in onset, and not necessarily similar in prognosis. With Fetal Alcohol Syndrome (FAS), the cause is known: chronic maternal alcoholism. The diagnostic picture is relatively clear, particularly in the early years, and the natural history is being documented. Furthermore, partial manifestations, probably associated with variations in dose, timing, conditions of exposure, and individual differences in sensitivity, are now being recognized. While FAS is a clearly defined entity, "suspected" or "partial" Fetal Alcohol Effects (FAE) can cover a wide range of disabilities and aberrations whose relationship with prenatal alcohol exposure can only be inferred. This paper will briefly review the historical perspective of alcohol teratogenesis, the identification of children with FAS and FAE, and implications for the fields of mental retardation and developmental disabilities. Preliminary data are presented from a new follow-up study of 38 adolescents and adults with FAS.

HISTORICAL PERSPECTIVE ON ALCOHOL TERATOGENESIS

Since early times there have been cautions and speculations about the dangers of alcohol use and abuse during pregnancy. (The reader is

---

This work was supported by a contract from the Indian Health Service, #240-83-0035, by grant number AA01455-11 from the National Institute of Alcohol Abuse and Alcoholism, by grants from the University of Washington Alcohol and Drug Abuse Institute and the Safeco Insurance Company. We gratefully acknowledge the assistance of Sandra P. Randels and Anne Garing.

referred to Warner & Rosett, 1975, and Streissguth & Martin, 1983, for more detailed accounts.) One of the first well-documented studies was carried out in 1899 by W. C. Sullivan, a physician at the Liverpool Jail in England, who found that female "drunkards" had two and one-half times the neonatal mortality as their nonalcoholic female relatives. However, such studies seem to have had little impact on medical practice and, as late as 1942, E. M. Jellinek, a physician internationally renowned for his work on alcoholism, reflected the prevalent view of the times, that the difficulties observed in the children of alcoholic parents resulted from the tumultuous family environment (Haggard & Jellinek, 1942).

In 1968, Paul Lemoine, a pediatrician in Nantes, France, published his studies on 120 children of alcoholic parents, noting a pattern of growth deficiency, malformations, and behavioral disturbances that seemed particularly characteristic in children whose mothers were alcoholic (Lemoine, Harousseau, Borteyru, & Menuet, 1968). Dr. Lemoine felt these characteristics were so specific that the alcoholism of the mothers could be suspected from the faces of their infants. Unfortunately, this work was published only in a local medical journal in France, where it remained untranslated and internationally unknown. In 1973, Jones, Smith, and colleagues published two papers in the *Lancet* describing independent observations of a similar pattern of malformations and growth deficiency in 11 children of alcoholic mothers; this work received immediate international interest (Jones & Smith, 1973; Jones, Smith, Ulleland, & Streissguth, 1973). Jones and Smith coined the term *Fetal Alcohol Syndrome* and clinical reports from many countries appeared. In the intervening 12 years, there have been over 2,000 scientific papers published on alcohol and pregnancy according to the National Clearinghouse on Alcohol Information of the National Institute of Alcohol Abuse and Alcoholism (NIAAA). Alcohol is now recognized as a teratogenic drug and Fetal Alcohol Syndrome is now a well-recognized cause of mental retardation.

PREVALENCE ESTIMATES

FAS is thought to be the third most prevalent known cause of mental retardation. Only Down syndrome and spina bifida are more prevalent. But, unlike Down syndrome, FAS cannot be diagnosed from a single laboratory test and, unlike spina bifida, there may be no flagrant physical marker at birth. To the untrained eye, the young infant with FAS may be just another growth deficient baby. The trained observer, on the other hand, will notice a cluster of subtle but specific characteristic facial features, the presence of growth deficiency, and some central nervous system problems that will help delineate the diagnosis. Nevertheless, because diagnosis in both newborn and child rests on a clinical judgment along with the presence of a positive history of maternal alcohol abuse during pregnancy, it is unlikely that reliable prevalence figures will be easy to obtain.

Systematic studies of newborns in three cities, conducted by clinicians experienced in diagnosing FAS, have yielded prevalence figures in the range of 1 in 750 live births (Dehaene et al., 1981, in Roubaix, France; Hanson, Streissguth, & Smith, 1978, in Seattle, Washington; and Olegård et al., 1979, in Göteborg, Sweden). Other studies have reported either lower figures (Sokol, Miller, & Reed, 1980) or higher figures (May, Hymbaugh, Aase, & Samet, 1983, in a study of American Indian tribes of the Southwest United States). The prevalence of FAS is a function of the drinking habits of women of childbearing age in the population and the skill and experience of the local diagnosticians. Unlike spina bifida and other major birth defects, FAS is very difficult to detect retrospectively from delivery records because the subtle diagnostic features are frequently overlooked in the newborn nursery. Likewise, the alcoholic mother may not be readily identified in the delivery room unless she meets the classic stereotype of the skid row alcoholic.

We suspect that there are large variations in the prevalence of FAS among different populations. May et al. (1983), for example, estimated that the prevalence of FAS ranged from 1 in 100 births on some Indian reservations to 1 in 750 on others. While it is possible that population differences in sensitivity to alcohol exist, a more likely explanation might be found in the drinking habits of the higher risk groups.

FAS has been diagnosed in children of all racial backgrounds born to mothers imbibing all kinds of alcoholic beverages. According to our personal communications, mothers of children with FAS tend to drink beer in Roubaix (a beer-producing region of France); white wine in Nantes (a white-wine-producing region); rum in the Reunion Isles (where rum is produced); and a mixture of beverages in many places such as Seattle. Regional studies can therefore be misleading. What seem to be differential prevalence figures for certain beverages more likely reflect regional beverage preferences and actual intake.

Unfortunately, there have been almost no systematic studies estimating the prevalence of FAS or maternal alcoholism among groups of retarded persons. This lack may be largely attributable to the extreme difficulty of conducting retrospective studies of maternal drinking habits. However, in 1981 Hagberg and colleagues published a report on the causes of mild mental retardation among school children 8 to 12 years of age in the city of Göteborg in Sweden (Hagberg, Hagberg, Lewerth, & Lindberg, 1981). Using a very strict definition of FAS and depending on retrospective reports of maternal alcoholism, this careful study found that 8% of the children classified as having mild mental retardation (IQ 50 to

70) had stigmata compatible with FAS and a maternal history of heavy drinking. The importance of this 8% figure is accentuated by the 5% figure for all known genetic causes of mild mental retardation in this study and the finding that 55% of the mildly retarded children were classified as *etiology unknown*. It may be many more years before the full impact of prenatal alcohol exposure on the cognitive, intellectual, and academic functioning of children is understood because of problems in evaluation of both the exposure and the outcome.

ALCOHOL AS A TERATOGEN

Teratogenic substances are those known to cause adverse effects on offspring as a result of gestational exposure. Teratogenic endpoints include death, malformation, growth deficiency, and functional effects (Wilson, 1977). In Figure 1, from Vorhees (1986), one can see that for those teratogens that cause all four types of teratogenic outcomes: (a) there is a dose/response curve for *each* outcome and (b) there is a dose/effects relationship among outcomes, so that the dose required to produce the different effects also varies. (For example, a higher dose is required to produce malformations than that needed to produce growth deficiency.) One can see then from Figure 1, which was derived from animal studies of many types of teratogens, that functional outcomes can be produced at lower levels of exposure than those producing malformations and growth deficiency.

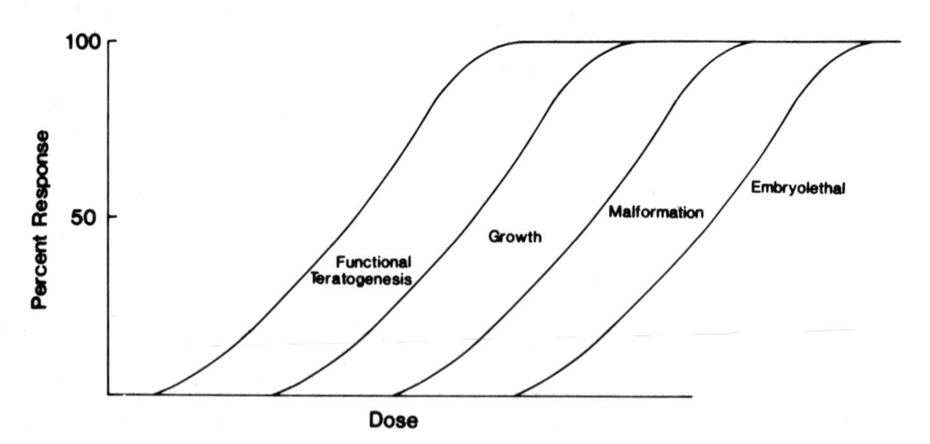

FIGURE 1: Idealized dose/response curves for the major manifestations of teratogenesis. The slope and spacing of the curves are dependent on the agent under investigation. The positions of the curves are only valid in their ordinal relationship to one another and if and only if the agent in question is capable of producing all four types of embryotoxicity shown. (From Vorhees, 1986.)

Teratogenically induced functional deficits have usually been defined in terms of the Central Nervous System (CNS). Functional effects on the hypothalamic-pituitary-adrenal pathway and the hypothalamic-pituitary-gonadal pathway are presently being explored in rodent studies with respect to prenatal alcohol exposure (Taylor, Nelson, Branch, Kokka, & Poland, 1984; Van Thiel, Parker, Udani, & Gavaler, 1984). One of the virtues of research on laboratory animals is that the dose/response relationship can be clearly established, even with behavioral endpoints. With human beings, in whom behavior is so multidetermined and exposure is so imprecisely measured, it is more difficult to relate specific functional effects to certain levels of exposure. Such difficulties arise particularly in the absence of physical findings (such as malformations and prenatally induced growth deficiency) that serve as markers of prenatal insult to the developing embryo and fetus. Thus in the individual case, we can be relatively more certain of the causal link to maternal alcoholism in FAS than in instances of *suspected Fetal Alcohol Effects,* particularly when the latter effects are primarily behavioral.

Prenatal alcohol exposure can produce all four teratogenic endpoints shown in Figure 1. In human beings we see an increased risk of spontaneous abortions, stillbirths, malformation, growth deficiency, and CNS effects related to prenatal alcohol exposure. (See Abel, Randall, & Riley, 1983, and Streissguth, Landesman-Dwyer, Martin, & Smith, 1980, for reviews of the literature.) Research on laboratory animals (where various factors such as nutrition, postnatal environment, and other exposures can be controlled) have clearly indicated that alcohol is teratogenic. (See Abel, 1982, and Randall, 1977, for reviews.) Typical findings from animal studies of alcohol teratogenesis include face and limb malformations, resorptions, decreased litter size, and growth deficiency. CNS effects have been frequently observed, particularly hippocampal effects, cerebellar effects, and changes in size and weight of the brain. (See CIBA Foundation, 1984, and West, 1986, for recent reviews.) Animal research on the behavioral teratology of alcohol has in general replicated the human findings with increased offspring activity, developmental delay, poor suckling, poor response inhibition, and decreased learning (Meyer & Riley, 1986).

As with other teratogens, however, not all exposed offspring are affected. Chernoff (1980) first demonstrated this for alcohol with experiments on several strains of mice. He showed that those with slow rates of alcohol metabolism had offspring with more abnormalities and growth deficiency than those with rapid alcohol metabolism. Not only do differences in maternal sensitivity affect the degree of damage, but offspring sensitivity plays a role as well. In animal studies, not all offspring are uniformly affected. Human dizygotic twins of alcoholic mothers are also often differentially affected, sometimes to the point of one being mentally retarded while the other is not. Their different genetic backgrounds apparently result in dissimilar sensitivity to equivalent gestational alcohol exposure.

Not all children born to alcoholic mothers will have FAS or even FAE. Estimates of the proportion of affected children vary according to the severity of the diagnosed condition and the severity of the maternal alcoholism. In an early study of chronically alcoholic, lower socioeconomic-class mothers, Jones, Smith, Streissguth, and Myrianthopoulis (1974) reported a 32% risk of FAS, using data from medical records from the National Perinatal Collaborative Study. Olegård et al. (1979) reported a 33% prevalence rate of FAS among alcoholic mothers and a 75% rate for partial effects. Majewski, Bierich, and Seidenberg (1978) reported a 43% prevalence among the most severely alcoholic mothers and a 20% prevalence among women with milder alcoholism. We estimate that perhaps one-third of the children born to chronic alcoholic mothers will have diagnosable FAS. Perhaps twice that many will have some fetal effects of alcohol.

Thus we can see that although alcohol is a teratogen, gestational exposure does not always result in damage to the offspring. The individual genetic factors that contribute to differential vulnerability in the individual case are not well understood at this time.

FETAL ALCOHOL SYNDROME: DIAGNOSTIC CONSIDERATIONS

Unlike Down syndrome or Turner syndrome, where laboratory tests provide a definitive diagnosis, FAS is diagnosed by clinical symptoms. The diagnosis rests on the clinical acuity of the diagnostician and the criteria used. Because full Fetal Alcohol Syndrome represents the end of a continuum of effects, apparent differences in outcome can occur depending on where the continuum is terminated. First, we will discuss the full syndrome.

A diagnosis of FAS is warranted when a child has a cluster of three characteristics: growth deficiency, certain dysmorphic features, and some CNS effects. The facial characteristics in FAS (Figure 2) include short palpebral fissures (eye slits), low nasal bridge, epicanthic folds, short nose, indistinct philtrum (the ridges running between the nose and the mouth), narrow upper lip, small chin, and flat midface. Other eye anomalies, such as ptosis (drooping eyelids) and strabismus (crossed eyes), have been noted with increased frequency, as have malformations of the external ear. Although many of these features occur in normal persons, it is the *cluster* of characteristics that is diagnostically important

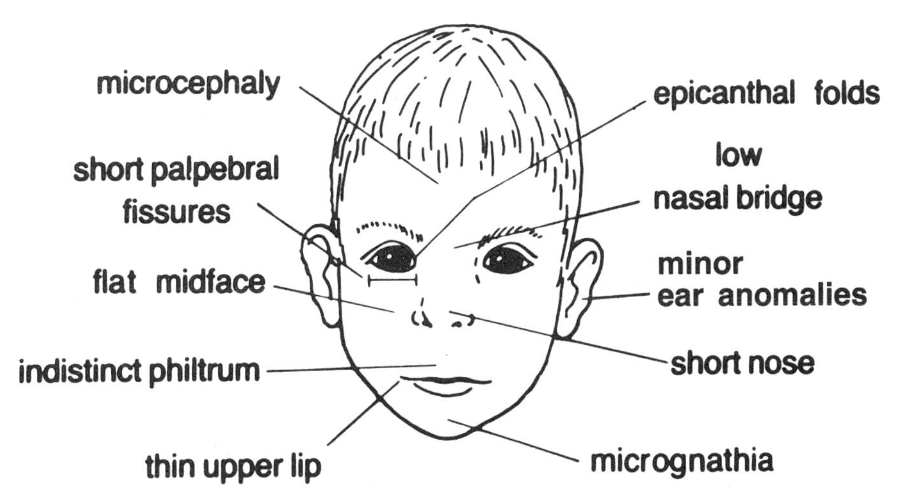

FIGURE 2: Common facial characteristics seen in children having Fetal Alcohol Syndrome. The characteristics on the left side are those most frequently seen in Fetal Alcohol Syndrome. Those on the right side are less specific. From Little & Streissguth (1982).

for FAS. Joint anomalies (particularly radio-ulnar synostosis), altered palmar crease patterns, and minor genital anomalies have also been reported in 26–50% of the patients. Heart defects occur in approximately 30–40% of children with FAS. Congenital eye defects (including optic nerve hypoplasia) have been recognized in 49% of the patients with FAS recently evaluated by Stromland (1985). (See Jones & Smith, 1975; Clarren & Smith, 1978; Clarren, 1981; and Majewski, 1981, for fuller descriptions of the phenotype in the Fetal Alcohol Syndrome.)

The growth deficiency typical of FAS is of prenatal onset and postnatal catch-up growth for height and head circumference generally does not occur. Children with FAS are usually below the third percentile in height, weight, and head circumference. As they develop, the reduced adipose tissue becomes more pronounced and as children they are often very thin. The pubescent and adult phenotype is now being recognized as different, however, and these differences will be discussed later.

CNS effects include retarded mental and motor development and a variety of developmental delays and learning difficulties, as well as tremulousness, hyperactivity, and poor attention spans. Small brain size and brain malformations (Figure 3) have been noted at autopsy, as well as abnormal migration of neural and glial cells out over the surface of the brain (Clarren, Alvord, Sumi, Streissguth, & Smith, 1978; Clarren, 1986). Abnormal electroencephalogram patterns in newborns and children with FAS have been noted and recent work has indicated that these are related specifically to alcohol abuse and not to smoking, that they persist during the newborn period, and that they are also observed in infants without FAS who are born to alcohol abusing mothers (Havlicek, Childiaeva, & Chernick, 1977; Chernick, Childiaeva, & Ioffe, 1983; Ioffe, Childiaeva, & Chernick, 1984).

FAS has been diagnosed in infants, children, adolescents, and adults. In the newborn infant the facial characteristics and growth deficiency have been the primary diagnostic criteria, although a variety of functional

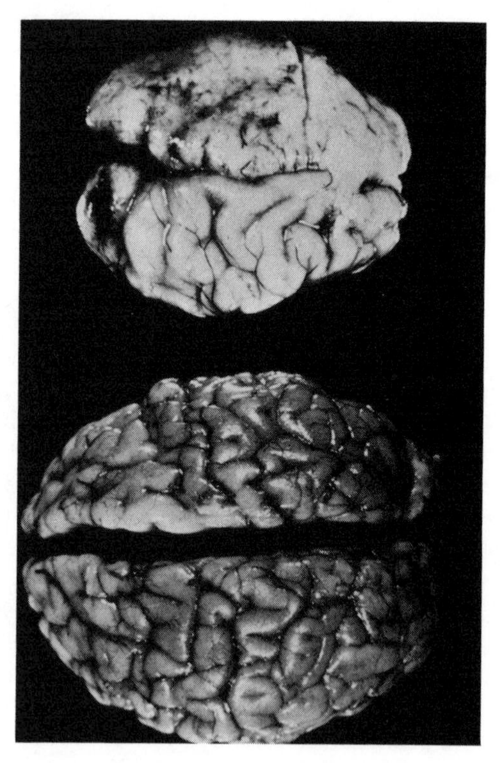

FIGURE 3: Comparison of the brain of a normal newborn with the brain of an infant with FAS who died 5 days after birth (Photograph courtesy of S. Clarren). Note the small size of the brain from the infant with FAS and that the gyral pattern is obscured by a leptomeningeal neuroglial heterotopia. From Streissguth, Landesman-Dwyer, Martin, & Smith (1980).

deficits have also been noted, including tremulousness, hypotonia, hyperactivity, hyperacusis (heightened sensitivity to sound), and opisthotonus (Jones & Smith, 1973; Pierog, Chandavasu, & Wexler, 1977). Weak sucking ability and other feeding difficulties, failure to thrive, and delayed development are also characteristic during the first year of life. In some instances, the microcephaly will be more marked at 9 to 12 months than at birth; this factor accounts for some failure to recognize FAS in newborn infants. However, the newborn profile can be particularly diagnostic with a short upturned nose, a convex philtral area, and small receding chin. Lemoine described this profile first in 1968 (Lemoine et al., 1968) and more recently, using many illustrations (Lemoine, 1985).

While recognition of FAS in infancy and childhood is fairly well established, the adolescent phenotype may not be so easily recognized. We have recently reported a 10-year follow-up study on the first 11 patients diagnosed with FAS in 1973 (Streissguth, Clarren, & Jones, 1985) as a first step in studying adolescents with FAS. As Figure 4 illustrates, some girls with FAS appear to take on more body fat around the time of menstruation. Because menarchy generally occurs with normal timing or earlier in girls with FAS, the female phenotype seems to change in early adolescence. Added body fat in the presence of short stature gives the pubescent girls with FAS a short, stocky appearance. However, this is not

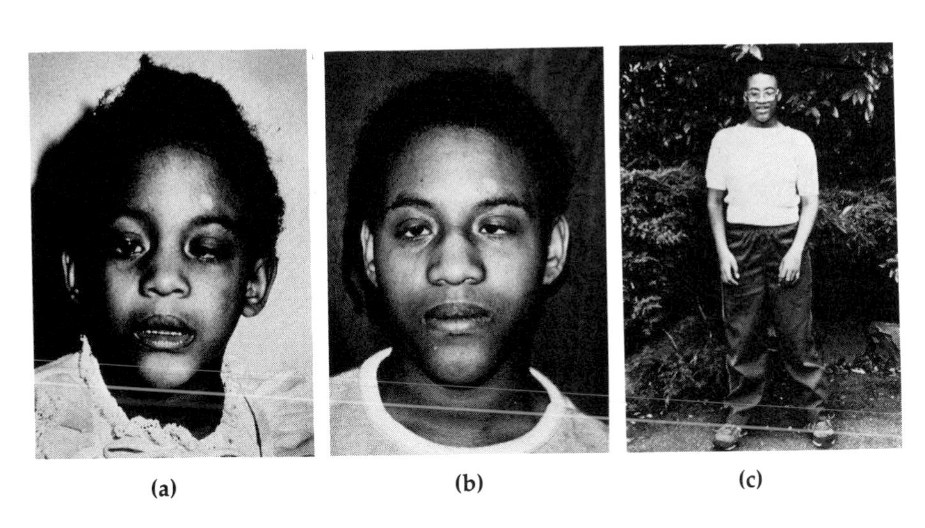

(a) (b) (c)

FIGURE 4: Patient at ages (a) 3 years 9 months and (b, c) 14 years 2 months. Note the persistence across ages of the short palpebral fissures, hypoplastic philtrum, strabismus, and ptosis; the increased growth of the nose and mandible; and the short, stocky stature often associated with puberty in girls with FAS. From Streissguth, Clarren, & Jones (1985).

always the case, and one certainly does see adolescent girls with FAS who remain thin. For boys with FAS, we have the impression that pubertal changes may be somewhat delayed, although this is still under investigation. Most adolescent boys with FAS that we have seen remain short and thin. Figure 5 shows a typical boy with FAS at 2 years of age and again at age 12. In adolescence and adulthood, short stature is often a noteworthy characteristic, particularly in the most severely affected individuals. However, genetic differences can contribute to normal stature in some patients.

Individual patients with FAS remain growth deficient into adolescence if one plots them against the norms, as Figure 6 indicates. However, it is clear from Table 1 that their weight-for-height age changes dramatically with puberty. We believe that the growth statistic that best summarizes the age changes in patients with FAS is the weight-for-height age. Table 1 demonstrates that the young patients, who are short and skinny, have very low weight-for-height age, while pubescent girls, who are short and stocky, have high weight-for-height ages. We believe that this changing pubescent phenotype may be one reason for the infrequent diagnosis of FAS among adolescents. Another reason may be the sketchiness of the maternal alcohol history 15 years after delivery, particularly among children who do not remain with their biologic parents.

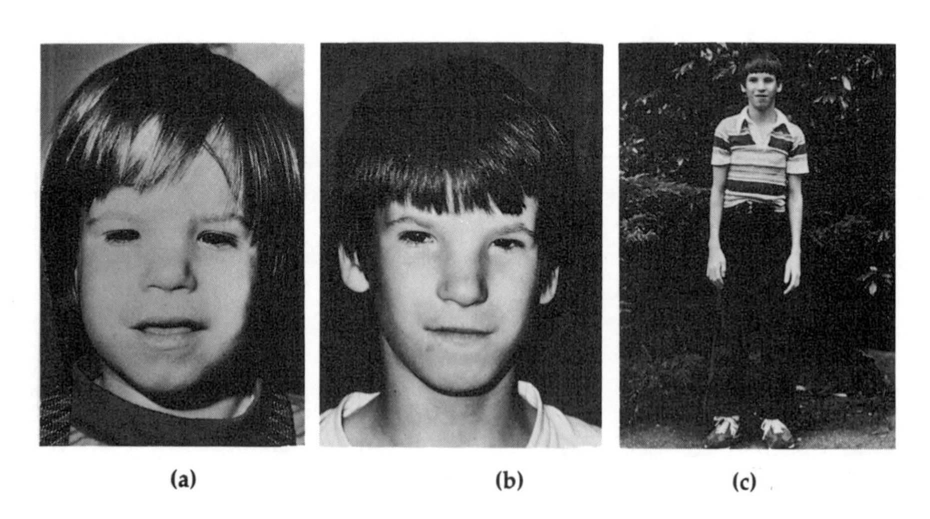

(a) (b) (c)

FIGURE 5: Patient 8 at ages (a) 2 years 6 months and (b, c) at 12 years 2 months. Note the short palpebral fissures, epicanthal folds, flat midface, hypoplastic philtrum, and thin upper vermillion border. Note also the short, lean prepubertal stature characteristic of young adolescent boys with FAS. From Streissguth, Clarren, & Jones (1985).

TABLE 1

Weight-for-Height Age at Three Different Ages: Original FAS Children

	PATIENT NO.	PRESCHOOL 1.5–5 YEARS	PREPUBERTAL 9–10	13–14 YRS	PUBERTY 13–14 YEARS
Boys	11	7.5%	5%	—	62%*
	4	15 %	37%	—	85%*
	7	8 %	50%	—	50%*
	3	5 %	15%	—	82%*
	2	15 %	38%	—	—
Girls	9	3.5%	17%	—	—
	8	3.5%	10%	20%	—
	6	<1%	10%	17%	—

Note: Height age represents chronological age on the growth charts at which the child's actual height fell at the 50th percentile (growth charts from National Center for Health Statistics, National Institutes of Health).
Weight-for-height age is the percentile at which the child's actual weight fell when plotted against the height age.
Girls and boys have been rank-ordered separately by severity of dysmorphology.
From Streissguth, Clarren, & Jones, 1985.
*Menarchy

It is important to note that the characteristic facial phenotype of FAS was determined from working with children from birth to 9 years. With puberty we see increased growth of the chin and nose (Figure 4), which can give the face quite a different appearance. In establishing the diagnosis of FAS in pubescent adolescents, it will be important to keep these changes in the facial phenotype in mind. In addition, one should not forget the other characteristics that also contribute to the diagnosis, such as earlier history of heart defects, minor hand anomalies (including altered palmar creases, hypoplastic nails, clinodactyly, camptodactyly, etc.), and radioulnar synostosis. (See Smith et al., 1981, for a review of radiographic findings in FAS.) Malformed, malaligned teeth are frequently noted in adolescents with FAS unless major orthodontics has been undertaken. Myopia and residual hearing loss from earlier otitis media are observed with increased frequency in later childhood and early adolescence (Streissguth et al., 1985).

The recognition of FAS in adulthood has not been well described in the literature, but we have been following a number of such patients in our clinic. Short stature seems characteristic of both males and females and increased adipose tissue is often noted in males between the ages of 20 and 30. Small head circumference seems more conspicuous with the mature body. Figures 7 & 8 show adult males with FAS photographed at different ages. We sometimes find that photographs of patients at earlier

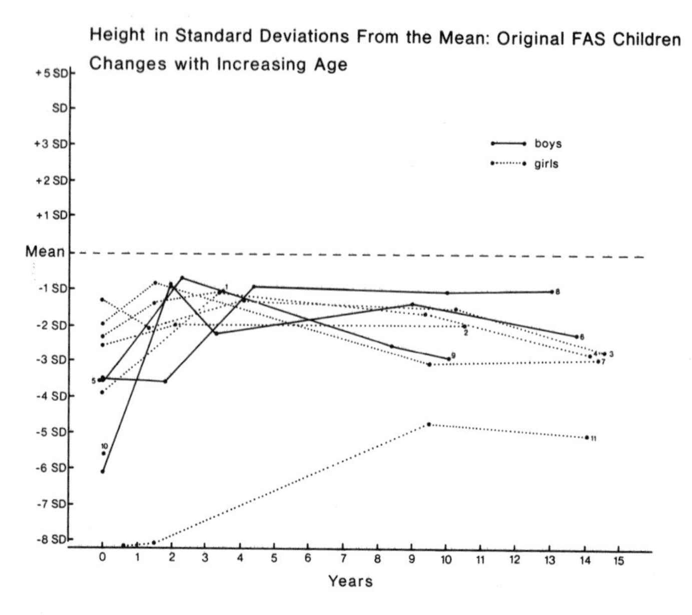

FIGURE 6a: Height curves with age. Records taken at five ages are plotted when available. From Streissguth, Clarren, & Jones (1985).

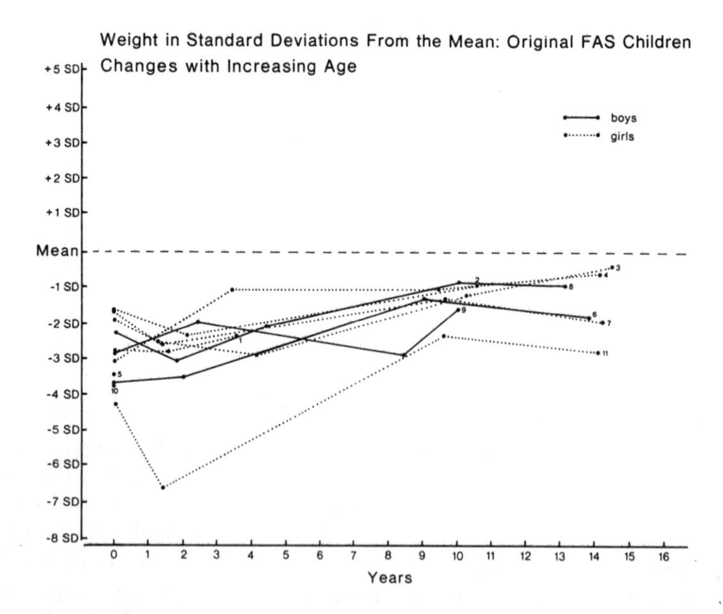

FIGURE 6b: Weight curves with age. Records taken at five ages are plotted when available. From Streissguth, Clarren, & Jones (1985).

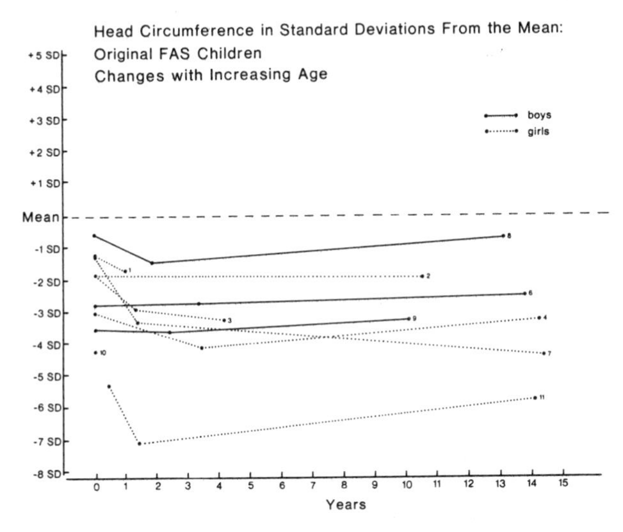

FIGURE 6c: Head circumference curves with age. Records taken at five ages are plotted when available. From Streissguth, Clarren, & Jones (1985).

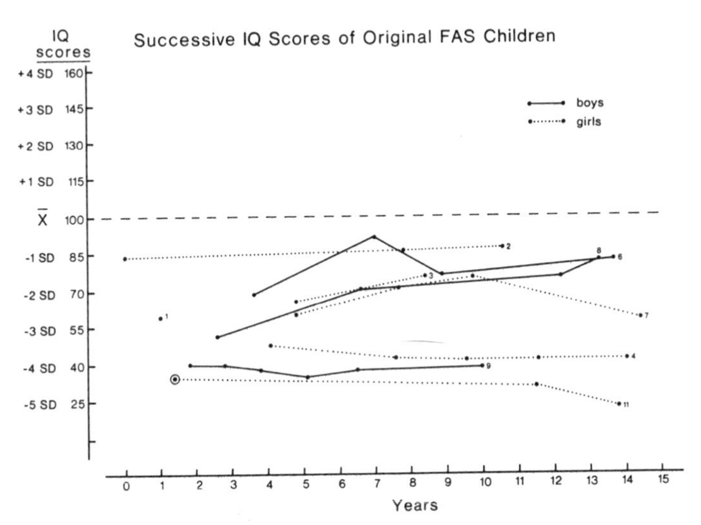

FIGURE 6d: IQ curves with age. Records taken at five ages are plotted when available. IQ scores are derived from individual age-appropriate tests of general intelligence and mental development, including the Wechsler Intelligence Scale for Children (revised), the Wechsler Preschool and Primary Scale of Intelligence, the Stanford-Binet Intelligence Scale Form L-M, and the Bayley Scales of Mental Development. The Stanford-Binet IQ scores reported have been recalculated according to norms published since then. The first IQ point for patient 11 is circled because it was measured from the Vineland Social Maturity Scale and clinical observation. From Streissguth, Clarren, & Jones (1985).

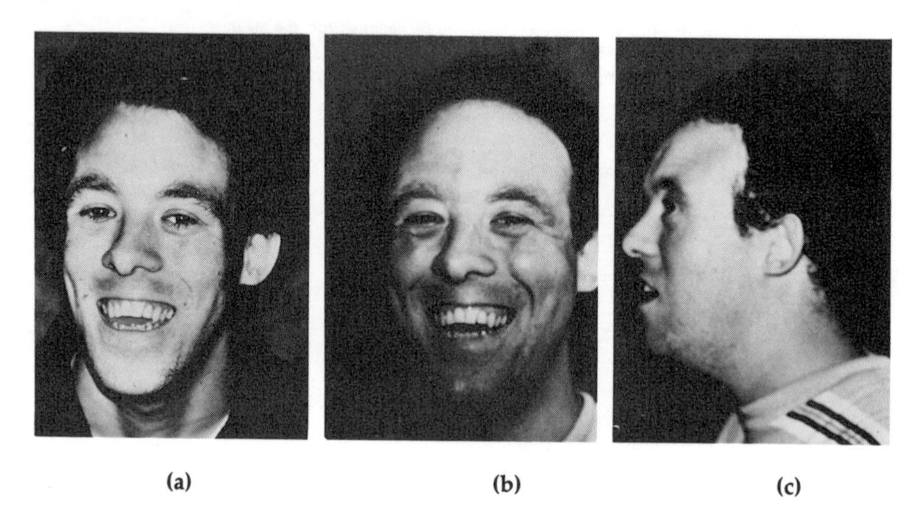

(a) (b) (c)

FIGURE 7: Adult male with FAS photographed at ages (a) 22 and (b, c) 28. Note the elongation of the chin with increasing age. The primary FAS facial anomalies of small palpebral fissures, smooth philtrum, and thin upper vermillion border are still present in the adult face.

ages (preferably 2 to 9 years) and early growth data are useful in establishing the diagnosis in adults. As with adolescents, it is important to consider the other phenotypic characteristics and not rely solely on facial

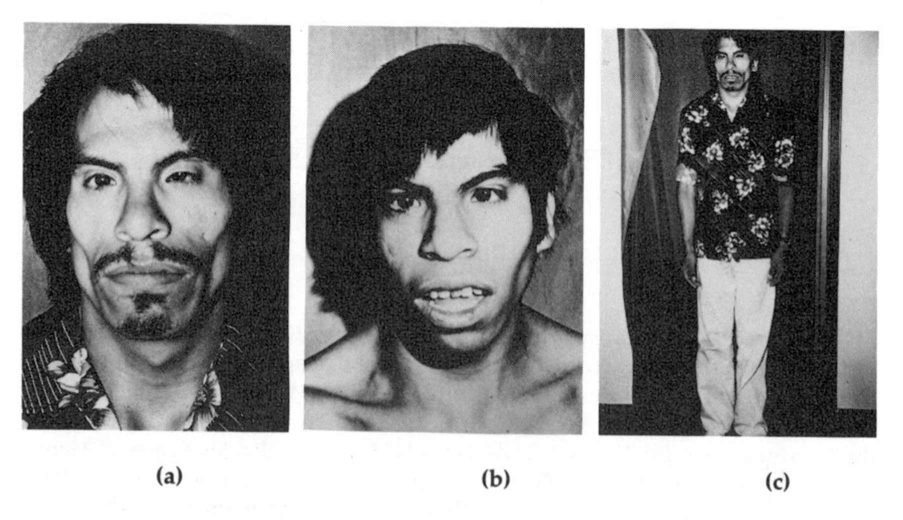

(a) (b) (c)

FIGURE 8: Adult male with FAS photographed at age 19 (a) and (b, c) 30. Note the long arms, the short, lean stature, and the poor posture.

features. In patients of all ages, diagnosis rests on the presence of growth retardation, a pattern of dysmorphic characteristics, and CNS effects. Further study of older patients is still necessary to clarify the adult phenotype and the relative importance of early growth deficiency in patients who have achieved maturity. Our studies of older patients thus far have suggested that the CNS effects may be the most enduring and the most significant.

FETAL ALCOHOL EFFECTS OR PARTIAL OR QUESTIONABLE FETAL ALCOHOL SYNDROME

All clinicians working with patients having FAS have appreciated the varying degrees of severity in affected patients. Full FAS is recognized as the far end of a continuum of effects and general agreement exists about FAS as a diagnostic entity, at least in the pre-adolescent child.

Classification of the "lesser" effects, however, has been far from systematic. Dehaene and colleagues in France (1977) and Majewski in Germany (1981) developed a system of classification involving three levels of severity of FAS. Dehaene's criteria involved clinical judgments while Majewski developed a weighted point system with quantitative cutoffs. Olegård and colleagues (1979) use the term *Partial FAS*. In the third and most recent edition of his classic book, *Recognizable Patterns of Human Malformation* (1982), David W. Smith preferred the term *Fetal Alcohol Effects* (FAE) to cover the continuum of clinically recognizable offspring effects associated with maternal alcohol abuse. Clarren (1981) suggested that the term *possible fetal alcohol effects* be used in differential diagnosis between the full FAS and cases where the cluster of symptoms is inadequate for definitive syndrome identification.

INTELLECTUAL DEVELOPMENT IN FETAL ALCOHOL SYNDROME

Level of Functioning in Childhood

The average IQ scores of groups of patients with this diagnosis will vary according to the severity of diagnostic criteria employed. Furthermore, the wide variation in IQ scores within groups of patients with FAS makes definitive prognostications difficult in the individual case.

Streissguth, Herman, and Smith (1978a), reported on the IQ scores of 20 patients between the ages of 7 months and 21 years who were diagnosed as having FAS by Dr. David W. Smith. Their mean IQ of 65 was comparable to the average IQ of patients with FAS reported from France and Germany (Dehaene et al., 1977; Lemoine et al., 1968; Majewski, 1981).

Table 2 shows that the severity of the FAS diagnosis is inversely related to IQ. This early finding has been replicated frequently in our clinical observations as well as by many other clinicians working with such patients. One can also see from Table 2, however, that there is considerable variation in IQ scores even among children within a given severity classification. We conclude from these findings that, although severity of FAS diagnosis is a good general indicator of level of functioning, one should be cautious in making predictions in the individual case. A full psychological evaluation should certainly be part of the workup on any child suspected of having FAS, and such workups should be repeated at key ages. Specific recommendations will be discussed later in this chapter.

Changes Over Time

A follow-up study of 17 patients with FAS seen 1 to 3 years after their initial examinations (Streissguth, Herman, & Smith, 1978b) indicated that while mean IQ scores remained constant, some individual children changed considerably during that time. As Figure 6 shows, four of the 19 children changed more than one standard deviation (15 IQ points); on retest, two had improved while two had lower scores. These individual changes were not associated with changes in the home environment or time of initial test. Maximal shifts in IQ were associated with entry into school which McCall described as a *transition age,* when a child's IQ appears to be particularly unstable (McCall, Applebaum, & Hogarty, 1973).

We have recently published a 10-year follow-up (Streissguth et al., 1985) of the original 11 children on whom the diagnosis of FAS was first used in 1973 (Jones et al., 1973; Jones & Smith, 1973). We found that for

TABLE 2

IQ in 20 Children with Fetal Alcohol Syndrome A Clinical Sample[a]

SEVERITY OF DIAGNOSIS	(N)	MEAN IQ	RANGE OF IQ
Mild and very mild	(4)	82	60 to 105
Moderate	(6)	68	59 to 81
Moderately severe	(5)	58	15 to 89
Severe	(5)	55	41 to 69
Summary	(20)	65	15 to 105

[a]Data from Streissguth, Herman, & Smith, 1978a.

most of these patients IQ remained quite stable over the 10-year period (Figure 6). Although most children remained fairly stable, one young boy had a gradual 30-point rise in IQ over this period. This magnitude of change is to be expected in some individuals in test/retest IQ studies (McCall et al., 1973); however, IQ scores of retarded persons are usually more stable than scores of normal persons. Although we could see no direct relationship in our follow-up study with improved IQ scores accompanying improved environmental circumstances, we did note that marked hyperactivity during the preschool years may have masked the early intellectual capacity of the child whose IQ rose from 50 to 80 during the 10-year period. We are not suggesting that all hyperactive children with FAS will show such a change, however, as our most hyperactive child has always has IQ scores in the 40–45 range. We simply suggest that IQ scores of very hyperactive children may be less predictive of their own later IQ levels than IQ scores of nonhyperactive preschool children. We intend to address this question in subsequent studies; at the present time it is merely a clinical impression.

Level of Functioning in Adolescents and Adults

Other than a few case reports, there is little data available on the long-term outlook for patients with FAS. To address this question, we are conducting a large follow-up study of a group of adults and adolescents who had previously been diagnosed FAS or FAE. Data are presented here on the first 38 patients examined, who range in age from 12 to 40 years, with a mean chronological age of 17 years 6 months. This sample includes 31 patients with a diagnosis of FAS and 7 patients with a diagnosis of *questionable FAS or FAE*. The sample includes 7 urban American Indians, 18 reservation Indians, 10 whites, and 3 blacks. IQ scores from the Wechsler Intelligence Scale for Children-Revised (WISC-R) or the Wechsler Adult Intelligence Scale-Revised (WAIS-R), depending on the patient's age, reveal a mean Full Scale IQ of 68. (See Figure 9 for the IQ distribution, which ranges from 39–105.) From Figure 9 we can also see that the 7 patients without the full syndrome had somewhat higher IQ scores than those with the full syndrome. (Although the IQ tests were administered after the dysmorphology exam, it would be impossible to say that the diagnostician did not use his estimate of the patient's intelligence as a factor in arriving at the diagnosis.) Table 3 presents the mean and median IQ subtest scores for this sample.

Figures 10 and 11 compare the Performance and Verbal IQ scores for these same 38 subjects. We can see that these adolescent and adult patients perform better on performance than verbal scales and that this finding holds across the entire distribution. Mean verbal IQ was 63 for the

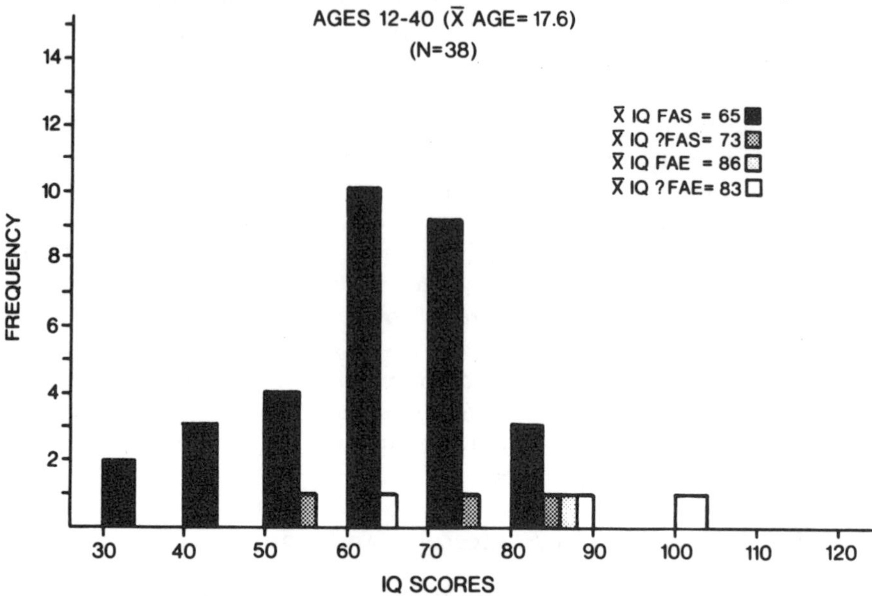

FIGURE 9: Frequency distribution of IQ scores for patients with Fetal Alcohol Syndrome and Fetal Alcohol Effects. The IQ range is 39–105. Note that the majority of patients fall in the 50–80 range, with a mean IQ of 68.

group; mean performance IQ was 77. Although there are no clear racial differences in overall IQ, the lower Verbal IQ scores of bilingual Indians may help account for the lower Verbal IQ of this sample.

The data from Figures 9, 10, and 11, as well as those presented in Figure 6, indicate that intellectual deficits persist among patients diagnosed with FAS, even into adolescence and adulthood. However, as in all clinical studies, the reader is cautioned not to over-generalize from these results. As ascertainment and follow-up bias can exist in clinical samples such as these, it is difficult to say to what extent these data are representative of all patients with FAS.

BEHAVIOR AND PERFORMANCE IN FETAL ALCOHOL SYNDROME

There are few systematic studies on behavioral and developmental problems in children with FAS, but two recent studies are relevant. In

TABLE 3

IQ Scores and Subtest Scores in 38 Adolescents and Adults with FAS and FAE

	MEAN	MEDIAN	RANGE
Full Scale IQ	67.97	69	39–105
Verbal IQ	63.29	77	39–88
Performance IQ	76.87	64	39–121
Information	3.18	2	1–9
Similarities	4.16	4	1–11
Arithmetic	3.82	3	1–10
Vocabulary	3.89	3	1–11
Comprehension	4.08	3	1–11
Digit span	4.4	4	1–9
Picture completion	7.21	7	1–14
Picture arrangement	5.87	6	0–15
Block design	6.55	7	1–12
Object assembly	7.71	8	1–14
Coding/digit symbol	5.16	4	1–13

Data from the FAS Follow-up Project, A.P. Streissguth, Department of Psychiatry and Behavioral Sciences, University of Washington School of Medicine, Seattle, WA.

1982, Steinhausen, Nestler, and Spohr described a group of 49 children with FAS who were between 3 and 15 years of age (mean age = 6). Because the mean IQ of this group was 89, the sample may have included more lightly affected children; diagnostic criteria are not discussed. Nevertheless, the authors systematically compared developmental problems and psychopathologic behaviors with a group of 28 controls matched in age, sex, socioeconomic status, and residence (i.e., biological parents and institutions). As Tables 4 and 5 indicate, there was a high percentage of developmental and psychopathologic symptoms associated with FAS.

A recent study from Sweden by Aronson, Olegård, and colleagues has described behavioral problems and performance deficits in 21 children of alcoholic mothers compared with controls matched for age, sex, birthweight, and gestational age. Half of the children were noted to have "malformations and/or other signs of FAS, and these children were consistently doing the most poorly." Children of alcoholic mothers not only were thinner, shorter, and had smaller head circumference on follow-up examination at almost 6 years (mean age), but they also had significantly poorer fine and gross motor performance and coordination when tested on a modified Oseretsky test (Kyllerman, Aronson, Sabel, Karlberg, Sandin, & Olegård, 1985).

In another report on this same study, Aronson, Kyllerman, Sabel, Sandin, and Olegård (1985) report the following results: The children of alcoholic mothers also had significantly lower IQ scores than the controls

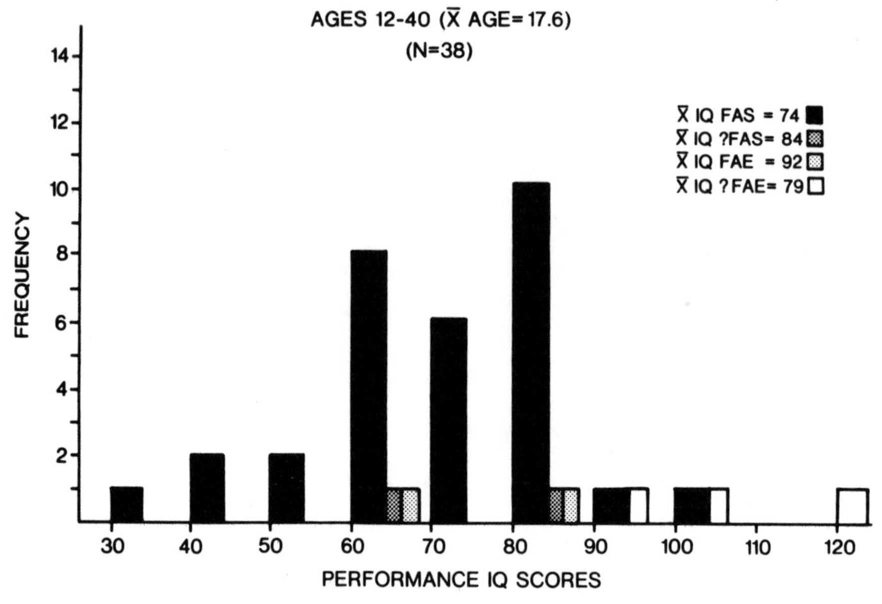

FIGURE 10: Frequency distribution of Performance IQ scores for patients with Fetal Alcohol Syndrome and Fetal Alcohol Effects. The range of Performance IQ scores is 39–121, with a mean of 77. Note how much higher the Performance IQ scores are than the Verbal IQ scores.

(IQ 95 vs. 112) and had significantly lower performance on all subscales of the Griffiths, with "practical reasoning" and eye-hand coordination being their lowest average areas of performance. On the Frostig Developmental Test of Visual Perception, half of the children of alcoholic mothers were

TABLE 4

Developmental Problems in FAS versus Control[a]

Neonatal complications	90%	32%
Problems with suck	70%	10%
Failure to thrive	90%	5%
Severe illness 1st year	65%	15%
Severe illness 2nd year	60%	16%
Retarded motor development	88%	16%
Retarded speech development	90%	22%
Retarded toilet training	70%	38%
Behavior disorders (preschool period)	50%	20%

[a]From Steinhausen, Nestler, and Spohr, 1982.
All differences significant at ≤.01, N = 49 FAS, 28 controls.

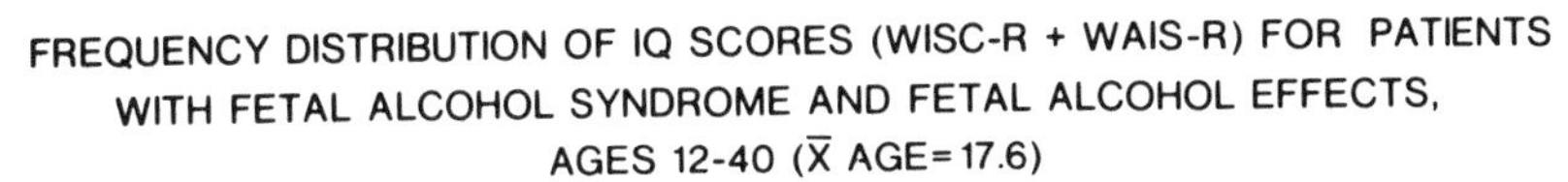

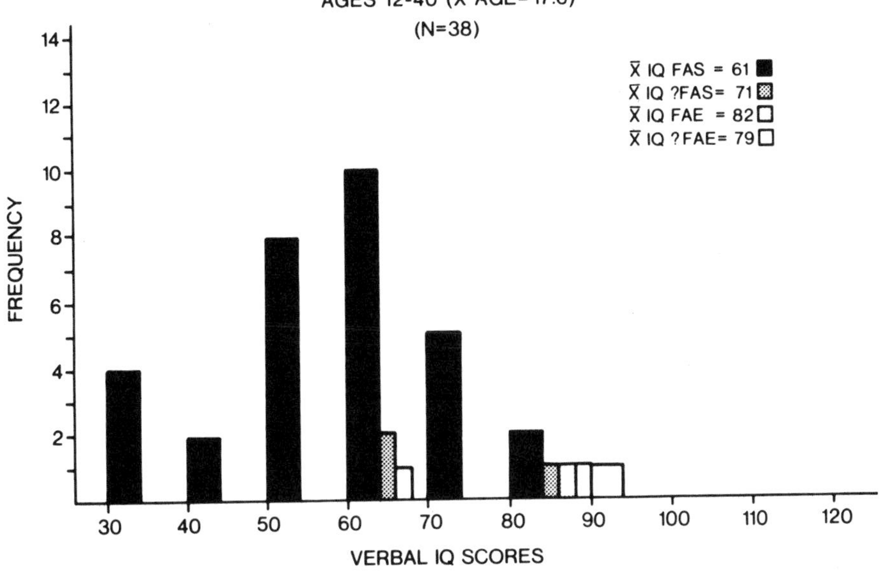

FAS Follow-up Study, 1985

FIGURE 11: Frequency distribution of Verbal IQ scores for patients with Fetal Alcohol Syndrome and Fetal Alcohol Effects. The mean Verbal IQ is 63 with a range of 39–88.

delayed by one year or more in perceptual development. On the Draw-a-Person Test, scored according to Koppitz, they had more signs of emotional instability irrespective of the caretaking arrangement, and over half were described as hyperactive, distractable, and having short attention spans. These behaviors are similar to those originally described by Lemoine in 1968.

From our own clinical experience, we believe that there is a behavioral phenotype of FAS that is as characteristic as the physical phenotype. At all ages, these patients are oriented toward social interactions and are outgoing. In young children with FAS, we note impulsivity, hyperactivity, poor attention spans, lack of inhibition, overfriendliness, overinquisitiveness, poor social judgment, poor sensitivity to social cues, excessive demands for physical contact and affection, and a sprightly, butterfly-like manner of movement. Fine motor problems are often noted, particularly in younger children; these include tremors, motor incoordination, or difficulty with eye-hand coordination. Slow performance time is noted as the children get

TABLE 5

Problems Occurring Significantly More Often in Children with Fetal Alcohol Syndrome When Compared with Matched Controls[a]

Problem
Hyperactivity
Outpatient therapy
Eating problems
Stutter/stammer
Reduced clarity of speech
Clumsiness: upper limbs
Rearing problems
Problems with peers
Strabismus
Clumsiness: lower limbs
Dependency
Hearing impairment
Abnormal habits
Reduced speech
Head and body rocking
Sleeping disturbance
Impaired concentration
Phobias

[a]From Steinhausen, Nestler, and Spohr, 1982.
Ordered by p value, from $p = <.0001$ to $<.05$; $N = 49$ FAS, 28 controls.

a little older, as though accomplishment of motor tasks requires extra effort. Difficulty remaining "on task" is noted across all ages.

As for all children, however, the predominant behavioral characteristics change as they mature. In infancy, the primary behaviors (in our clinical opinion) include weak suck and poor nursing, disrupted sleep patterns, poor habituation (failure to "tune out" repetitive stimulation, and consequent increasing responsiveness to repeated stimuli), and a low level of persistent focus on environmental stimuli. Absence of "stranger anxiety" and fearlessness in new social situations that would normally provoke a short period of appraisal are frequently noted in infants and young children with FAS.

During the preschool years, hyperactivity and extreme intrepidness are often noted. At this age their high activity level, their fearlessness, and their unresponsiveness to verbal cautions combine to make them particularly difficult to manage. Language development is often delayed, but seems to be less of a problem to parents because they tend to adjust their expectations in accordance with the children's small size. As speech emerges, articulation defects, echolalia, and perseveration are often noted, along with a shortness of sentences. Occasional long-term memory for some particular event often encourages parents to believe that mental development is, indeed, proceeding adequately, if a little slowly.

Difficulty with language comprehension is observed less frequently in a clinical sense than difficulty with language expression.

With the onset of school, hyperactivity continues to be a problem, although these children's general amicability and efforts to please can endear them to some teachers. Fine motor problems, particularly with graphic skills, and compounded by slow performance time, may delay learning in the primary grades. The more mildly affected children do respond favorably to tutoring and remedial help; after some initial difficulty they often attain an adequate grasp of reading and spelling, again an indication to their parents and teachers that progress is possible. In the primary grades, when one compares standard scores for reading and spelling with the children's standard scores for intelligence, they often seem to be overachievers. However, on a long-term basis, we have found that their IQ scores are ultimately better predictors of their later academic abilities than their early reading and spelling capabilities. As the more mildly affected children get older, spelling often stands out as their highest level of achievement. In terms of reading skill, their comprehension fails to keep pace with their word-recognition abilities. Arithmetic, in the first couple of grades, does not seem to present special problems (beyond those commensurate with their overall level of performance). However, memorization of the multiplication tables often presents a major stumbling block and, with increasing age, arithmetic skill falls progressively behind even in comparison to an individual child's own spelling and word-recognition skills.

Across all ages, children with FAS usually present the clinical appearance of being more intelligent than their IQ scores suggest. They also have a highly social orientation that keeps them directed toward the people in their environment. In benign environments, they can be initially charming, but are often overly intrusive, overly talkative, and overly close, in both a physical and a personal sense, to those around them.

As they get older and move into adolescence, school becomes increasingly difficult. Their poor social judgment and lack of impulse control often contribute to their loneliness and their having few friends. Adults and younger children are more frequent companions than peers. Problems with self-direction, decision-making, pursuing goals, and attaining independence become apparent with adolescence. Further studies of the special cognitive deficits of adults with FAS are urgently needed.

ADAPTIVE AND ACADEMIC FUNCTIONING IN FETAL ALCOHOL SYNDROME

Little systematic data are available on younger FAS patients with respect to adaptive functioning. In the original paper describing the first eight patients, we had Vineland Social Quotients on 4 of the 8 children; these were uniformly lower than both the IQ scores and the chronological age scores for these patients (Jones et al., 1973). The mean social quotient was 32 months; their mean chronological age was 42 months.

With our adolescent/adult follow-up sample, we have used the new Vineland Adaptive Behavior Scales. As Table 6 indicates, these patients have significant deficits in adaptive living skills. Although the group of patients for whom Vineland scores were available ranged from 12 to 24 years of age, only 2 of the 28 had an adaptive behavior level of 11 years or more. The mean chronological age of this group was 16½ years; however, their average adaptive behavior level was equivalent to that of most 9-year-olds. Their daily living skills were somewhat better, as Table 6 indicates, but socialization skills and communication skills were their poorest areas of performance. On the Peabody Picture Vocabulary Test, these patients had a mean receptive language age of 6½ years, despite a chronological age of 16½ years. Careful planning in the middle and high school years will be necessary to assure that they are equipped for life beyond the school years. Hopefully, with careful earlier diagnosis and

TABLE 6

Functional and Academic Deficits of Adolescents and Adults with FAS and FAE

Skill Measured/(Test Administered)	N	Chronological Age		Age or Grade Equivalent	
		Range	Mean	Mean	Range
VINELAND					
Adaptive Behavior Skills (Age equivalent)	29	12–24	16.6	9.1	(4.7–15.6)
Communication Skills (Age equivalent)	28	12–23	16.6	9.0	(4.0–15.9)
Daily Living Skills (Age equivalent)	28	12–24	16.6	10.10	(3.9–19.10)
Socialization Skills (Age equivalent)	29	12–24	16.6	7.5	(2.1–17.3)
PPVT					
Receptive Language (Age equivalent)	17	12–23	16.6	6.8	(3.0–13.9)
WRAT					
Reading (Word Recognition) (Grade equivalent)	37	12–40	17.7	4.11	(N.7–10.9)
Spelling (Grade equivalent)	37	12–40	17.7	4.3	(N.4–8.5)
Arithmetic (Grade equivalent)	37	12–40	17.7	3.0	(N.7–5.9)

Note: PPVT = Peabody Picture Vocabulary Test
VINELAND = Vineland Adaptive Behavior Scales
WRAT = Wide Range Achievement Test

Data from the FAS Follow-up Project, A.P. Streissguth, Department of Psychiatry and Behavioral Sciences, University of Washington School of Medicine, Seattle, WA.

planning, the next generation of patients with FAS will be better equipped for adaptive living.

Academic functioning of this group of adolescents and adults with FAS (Table 6) indicates that as a group they were fairly impaired, with reading and spelling skills at the 4th grade level and arithmetic skills at the 3rd grade level, as measured by the Wide Range Achievement Test (WRAT). Poor arithmetic skills seem characteristic of these patients, with only four of the 37 functioning at the 5th grade arithmetic level and none beyond. The implications of such low arithmetic scores coupled with the low Vineland Adaptive Behavior scores make the prospect for independent living seem somewhat ominous. Nevertheless, for reading and spelling there are some individuals whose skills are adequate. Six of the 37 adolescents and adults have spelling skills ranging from 6th through 8th grade; and 16 have reading skills ranging from the 5th through 8th grade level. Although one man of 39 years reads at the 10th grade level, in general those patients with better reading and spelling skills are the 13- to 15-year-olds. It is possible that this group will continue improving in these skill areas as they complete school. It is our clinical impression that comprehension lags behind word-recognition skills and that this gap increases with age. With these patients, a more meaningful reading score might be obtained from a reading comprehension test rather than the word recognition skills tested with the WRAT.

This chapter does not purport to be a literature review, but rather a summarization of our own clinical and empirical work on FAS over the past 12 years. We have recently written a chapter that is a thorough review of the literature on the behavioral teratology of alcohol up to 1985 (Streissguth, 1986a), and another chapter (Streissguth, 1986b), that reviews that literature on alcohol and smoking as causative factors in childhood learning disabilities. We would also like to refer the reader to several other papers on clinical aspects of FAS, including: Crepin and Dehaene (1980); Olegård et al. (1979); Majewski (1981); Steinhausen et al. (1982); Spohr and Steinhausen (1984); and Aronson et al. (1985). As is usual with new syndromes, the majority of the clinical papers describe the physical phenotype, while the behavioral phenotype is more poorly delineated. We expect that within the next 10-year period we will reach a more complete understanding of the full psychological import of this preventable form of mental retardation and developmental disability.

RECOMMENDATIONS FOR PREVENTION

Because FAS and FAE are preventable forms of mental retardation and developmental disability, the implications for primary prevention are clear. Anything that can be done to prevent or decrease maternal alcohol abuse during pregnancy should decrease the prevalence of FAS. Such actions can include public health recommendations such as the recommendation by the Surgeon General of the United States that women refrain from alcohol use during pregnancy (1981) and general policy statements of influential organizations cautioning against alcohol abuse during pregnancy such as the one by the American Medical Association (1983).

Campaigns to inform the public about the risks of drinking during pregnancy have been undertaken by many individual states, including Wisconsin, Michigan, South Carolina, North Carolina, Florida, and New York, to name a few. Media campaigns with TV, radio, and newspaper coverage have usually been supplemented with posters, brochures, bumper stickers, and bus signs. In New York City, official notices about the risk of birth defects must be posted in establishments serving alcoholic beverages.

Educational campaigns for in-service training of health care professionals and educators have also been carried out by many agencies for such groups as physicians, nurses, midwives, school teachers, occupational and physical therapists, speech and hearing specialists, and social workers. Experience in our own community suggests that in-service training and public education about the risks of drinking during pregnancy should be offered on a regular basis to meet ongoing needs.

Assessment of drinking during pregnancy and detection and help for pregnant women with alcohol problems are some of the critical needs in prevention of fetal alcohol effects. Rosett and Weiner have written extensively on this topic. (See Rosett, Weiner, and Edelin, 1981, for example.) The Fall 1985 issue of *Alcohol Health and Research World* is concerned entirely with FAS and preventing alcohol-related birth defects (Podolsky & Ronan, 1985). The reader is also referred to Little, Young, Streissguth, and Uhl (1984), which describes a demonstration program to prevent fetal alcohol effects. The program activities for this project included public education, professional training, volunteer services, a 24-hour crisis/telephone information line, adult treatment and education services (including those for pregnant women), and assessment services for children exposed prenatally to heavy doses of alcohol. Follow-up studies indicated that significantly more of the local population, the local pregnant women, and the local health professionals professed belief in abstinence from alcohol during pregnancy. Pregnant women with drinking problems who decreased their alcohol consumption during pregnancy had healthier infants. In terms of cost-effectiveness, this demonstration project cost about $1 million, approximately the cost of maintaining one severely retarded child for his or her lifetime.

RECOMMENDATIONS FOR INTERVENTION

Intervention work should focus on recognition of affected children so that they can be helped to develop to their own best potential. As alcoholic mothers are at high risk to produce another child with FAS after the first, indentification of one such child in a family may also be an important factor in prevention.

Diagnosis

Early diagnosis of the child with FAS is a key to proper care and case management. Ideally this diagnosis will be made at birth so that appropriate interventions can be undertaken immediately for the safety of mother and child. Because mothers who give birth to infants with FAS are at high risk themselves for alcohol-related morbidity and mortality, these families are often in need of intensive social service and public health supports. For affected infants, failure to thrive, pneumonia, child neglect, and abuse are some of the risks. Often foster and adoptive homes must be sought. Proper diagnosis in early infancy can facilitate placement.

Diagnosis during preschool years can assure proper educational planning for the child, including Headstart, and can facilitate entrance into the proper school setting. As in infancy, there may be a need for family support or for foster or adoptive placement.

Diagnosis during adolescence can facilitate proper planning for job training and adaptive living skills. In our experience the diagnosis, at whatever age it is made, is an important factor in proper management and recommendations. In patients with FAS this is particularly important because of the discrepancy between the rather alert verbal manner that many of these patients manifest and their generally poor level of attention and memory skills. Diagnosis should ideally be made by a pediatrician experienced in dysmorphology, but in many states genetics clinics are the best qualified to make the diagnosis. Even in the absence of a definitive diagnosis, we recommend considering children of alcoholic mothers as a group at risk. Thorough evaluation and follow-up should occur, particularly in the presence of any developmental delays or disabilities on the part of the child.

Case Management

The developmental work-up of the child with FAS should include several components:

1. A thorough physical examination with special emphasis on cardiac, orthopedic, sensory, and orthodontic problems, and nutrition. These represent the areas in which interventions are most frequently needed after infancy (Streissguth et al., 1985).

2. A thorough family history work-up to evaluate parental alcoholism (at the present and during pregnancy) and present living situation. Involvement with children's protective services, adoption and foster care agencies, and legal services is often necessary. Support services for families are often required, even for surrogate parents. These include public health support services, counseling, some form of respite care, and financial planning and placement for older patients. We have found that those patients placed in highly structured environments have done best.

3. A thorough psychological/educational/vocational work-up, including age-appropriate IQ and achievement tests, tests of receptive language and adaptive living skills, and appropriate behavior and problem checklists. Neuropsychological testing with particular emphasis on memory, problem solving skills, and attention can be helpful in establishing the particular pattern of deficit in the individual child.

We find that the generally adequate interpersonal skills and borderline IQ scores that many of these patients show in the early school years can mask their difficulties with problem solving, judgment, comprehension, and attention, all of which cause increasing problems as they mature.

Psychological/educational work-ups seem most important at certain key ages, including infancy, later preschool years, later primary grades, middle school, and during high school. From middle school onward we find these patients having increased difficulty with academic subjects. Therefore, at some point during the high school years we recommend assessment for possible vocational placement and development of daily living skills.

4. Vocational training and developmental disabilities evaluation become increasingly important as these patients mature. For many such patients an increased emphasis on vocational training, adaptive living skills, and satisfying work experiences will be necessary to bridge the gap into successful living as an adult. Management of money and time are two important skills for which early training can be particularly helpful.

SUMMARY

Fetal Alcohol Syndrome (FAS) and Fetal Alcohol Effects (FAE) are preventable forms of mental retardation and developmental disability caused by heavy prenatal alcohol exposure. Our best evidence of the overall prevalence of FAS is around 1 in 750 live births, but this figure will vary according to the drinking habits of the community and the diagnostic skills and interests of local physicians. It is likely that many infants are born with FAS or FAE, are never recognized as such, and are never properly diagnosed or evaluated. Other diagnoses that are sometimes confused with FAS include Noonan syndrome and William syndrome. More often, children with milder FAS or FAE go unrecognized. Careful evaluation of possible maternal alcohol abuse during pregnancy can be an important factor in differential diagnosis and proper case management.

Alcohol is a teratogenic drug that can produce a wide variety of deficits from prenatal exposure, depending on the dose, timing, and conditions of exposure, as well as on individual differences in sensitivity on the part of the mother and the child. Not all children who are exposed are affected. Perhaps 30–40% of the children of chronic alcoholic mothers who were drinking during pregnancy will have FAS. These children are at high risk for mental retardation or developmental disability. Even within this group, however, there can be large individual differences in eventual outcome. Prognosis involves an interaction between the extent of the damage and the stability and structure of the environment. Children whose mothers were abusing alcohol during pregnancy can be at risk for various learning and attentional problems even without FAS, but in the absence of morphologic effects, the diagnostic and prognostic picture is less clear. Systematic efforts toward both prevention and intervention can assure that each child develops to his or her own best potential.

REFERENCES

Abel, E.L. (1982). *Fetal Alcohol Syndrome: Volume III: Animal studies.* Boca Raton, Florida: CRC Press, Inc.

Abel, E.L., Randall, C.L., & Riley, E.P. (1983). Alcohol consumption and prenatal development. In B. Tabakoff, P.B. Sutker, & C.L. Randall (Eds.), *Medical and social aspects of alcohol abuse.* New York: Plenum Press.

American Medical Association. (1983). Fetal effects of maternal alcohol use—Council Report from the Council on Scientific Affairs, Division of Scientific Analysis of Technology. *Journal of the American Medical Association, 249*(18), 2517–2531.

Aronson, M., Kyllerman, M., Sabel, K.G., Sandin, B., & Olegard, R. (1985). Children of alcoholic mothers: Developmental, perceptual and behavioural characteristics as compared to matched controls. *Acta Paediatrica Scandinavica, 74,* 27–35.

Chernick, V., Childiaeva, R., & Ioffe, S. (1983). Effects of maternal alcohol intake and smoking on neonatal electroencephalogram and anthropometric measurements. *American Journal of Obstetrics and Gynecology, 146*(1), 41–47.

Chernoff, G.F. (1980). The Fetal Alcohol Syndrome in mice: Maternal variables. *Teratology, 22,* 71–75.

CIBA Foundation Symposium No. 105. (1984). *Mechanisms of alcohol damage in utero.* London: Pitman.

Clarren, S.K. (1981). Recognition of Fetal Alcohol Syndrome. *Journal of the American Medical Association, 245,* 2436–2439.

Clarren, S.K. (1986). Neuropathology in the Fetal Alcohol Syndrome. In J.R. West (Ed.), *Alcohol and brain development.* New York: Oxford University Press, 1986.

Clarren, S.K., Alvord, E.C., Sumi, S.M., Streissguth, A.P., & Smith, D.W. (1978). Brain malformations related to prenatal exposure to ethanol. *Journal of Pediatrics, 92,* 64–67.
Clarren, S.K., & Smith, D.W. (1978). The fetal alcohol syndrome. *New England Journal of Medicine, 298,* 1063–1067.
Crepin, G., & Dehaene, P. (1980). Lè nouveau-ne de mere alcoolique, signes cliniques, devenir. *Dixiemes Journees Nationales.* Deauville.
Dehaene, P., Crepin, G., Delahousse, G., Querleu, D., Walbaum, R., Titran, M., & Samaille-Villette, C. (1981). Aspects epidemiologiques du syndrome d'alcoolisme foetal. *La Nouvelle Press Medicale, 10*(32), 2639–2643.
Dehaene, P., Samaille-Villette, P., Crepin, G., Walbaum, R., Deroubaix, P., & Blanc-Garin, A.P. (1977). Le syndrome d'alcoolisme foetal dans le nord de la France. *La Revue de L'alcoolisme, 23,* 145–158.
Hagberg, B., Hagberg, G., Lewerth, A., Lindberg, U. (1981). Mild mental retardation in Swedish school children II: Etiologic and pathogenic aspects. *Acta Paediatrica Scandinavica, 70,* 445–452.
Haggard, H.W., and Jellinek, E.M. (1942). *Alcohol explored.* New York: Doubleday.
Hanson, J.W., Streissguth, A.P., & Smith D.W. (1978). The effects of moderate alcohol consumption during pregnancy on fetal growth and morphogenesis. *Journal of Pediatrics, 92*(3), 457–460.
Havlicek, V., Childiaeva, R., & Chernick, V. (1977). EEG frequency spectrum characteristics of sleep states in infants of alcohol mothers. *Neuropadiatrie, 8*(4), 360–373.
Ioffe, S., Childiaeva, R., & Chernick, V. (1984). Prolonged effects of maternal alcohol ingestion on the neonatal electroencephalogram. *Pediatrics, 74,* 330–335.
Jones, K.L., & Smith, D.W. (1973). Recognition of the Fetal Alcohol Syndrome in early infancy. *Lancet, 2,* 999–1001.
Jones, K.L., & Smith, D.W. (1975). The Fetal Alcohol Syndrome. *Teratology, 12,* 1–10.
Jones, K.L., Smith, D.W., Streissguth, A.P., & Myrianthopoulos, N.C. (1974). Outcome in offspring of chronic alcoholic women. *Lancet, 1,* 1076–1078.
Jones, K.L., Smith, D.W., Ulleland, C.N., & Streissguth, A.P. (1973). Pattern of malformation in offspring of chronic alcoholic mothers. *Lancet, 1,* 1267–1271.
Kyllerman, M., Aronson, M., Sabel, K.G., Karlberg, E., Sandin, B., & Olegård, R. (1985). Children of alcoholic mothers: Growth and motor performance compared to matched controls. *Acta Paediatrica Scandinavica, 74,* 20–26.
Lemoine, P. (1985). The observations of 200 cases of fetal alcohol syndrome observed during 25 years: Some information of clinical and pathological interest. *Proceedings of the 34th International Congress on Alcoholism and Drug Dependence.* Alberta Alcohol and Drug Abuse Commission.
Lemoine, P., Harousseau, H., Borteyru, J.P., & Menuet, J.C. (1968). Les enfants de parents alcooliques. Anomalies observees. A propos de 127 cas. *Paris, Ouest Medical, 21,* 476–482.
Little, R.E., & Streissguth, A.P. (1982). Alcohol, pregnancy, and the Fetal Alcohol Syndrome. In *Alcohol Use and Its Medical Consequences: A Comprehensive Teaching Program for Biomedical Education.* Project Cork of Dartmouth Medical School. (Slide/teaching unit available from Milner-Fenwick, Inc., 2125 Greenspring Drive, Timonium, MD 21093.)
Little, R.E., Young, A., Streissguth, A.P., & Uhl, C.N. (1984). Preventing fetal alcohol effects: Effectiveness of a demonstration project. In M. O'Connor & J. Whelan (Eds.), CIBA Foundation Symposium #105: *Mechanisms of alcohol damage in utero* (pp. 254–274). London: Pitman.
Majewski, F. (1981). Alcohol embryopathy: Some facts and speculations about pathogenesis. *Neurobehavioral Toxicology and Teratology, 3,* 129–144.
Majewski, F., Bierich, J.R., & Seinenberg, J. (1978). The incidence and pathogenesis of alcohol embryopathy. *Monatsschrift Fur Kinderheilkunde, 126,* 284–285.
May, P.A., Hymbaugh, K.J., Aase, J.M., & Samet, J.M. (1983). Epidemiology of Fetal Alcohol Syndrome among American Indians of the Southwest. *Social Biology, 30*(4), 374–387.
McCall, R.B., Applebaum, M.I., & Hogarty, P.S. (1973). Developmental changes in mental performance. *Monographs of The Society for Research in Child Development,* Serial No. 150, *38*(3).

Meyer, P.A., & Riley, E.P. (1986). Behavioral teratology of alcohol. In E.P. Riley & C.V. Voorhees (Eds.), *Handbook of behavioral teratology*. New York: Plenum Press.

New York City, Department of Health. Warning: Drinking alcohol beverages during pregnancy can cause birth defects. *The City Council Local Law 63*.

Olegård, R., Sabel, K.G., Aronson, M., Sandin, B., Johansson, P.R., Carlsson, C., Kyllerman, M., Iversen, K., & Hrbek, A., (1979). Effects on the child of alcohol abuse during pregnancy. *Acta Paediatrica Scandinavica Supplement, 275*, 112–121.

Pierog, S., Chandavasu, O., & Wexler, I. (1977). Withdrawal symptoms in infants with the Fetal Alcohol Syndrome. *Journal of Pediatrics, 90*, 630–633.

Podolsky, D.M., & Ronan, L. (Eds.) (1985). Preventing alcohol-related birth defects [Special issue]. *Alcohol Health and World Research, 10*(1).

Randall, C.J. (1977). Teratogenic effects of in utero ethanol exposure. In K. Bloom (Ed.), *Alcohol and opiates: Neurochemical and behavioral mechanisms* (pp. 91–107). New York: Academic Press.

Riley, E.P., & Vorhees, C.V. (1986). *Handbook of behavioral teratology*. New York: Plenum Press.

Rosett, H.L., Weiner, L., & Edelin, K.C. (1981). Strategies for prevention of fetal alcohol effects. *Journal of Obstetrics & Gynecology, 57*, 1–7.

Smith, D.F., Sandor, G.G., MacLeod, P.M., Tredwell, S., Wood, B., & Newman, D.E. (1981). Intrinsic defects in the fetal alcohol syndrome: Studies on 76 cases from British Columbia and the Yukon Territory. *Neurobehavioral Toxicology and Teratology, 3*, 145–152.

Smith, D.W. (1982). *Recognizable patterns of human malformation (3rd ed.)*. Philadelphia: W.B. Saunder Co.

Sokol, R.J., Miller, S.I., & Reed, G. (1980). Alcohol abuse during pregnancy: An epidemiologic study. *Alcoholism: Clinical and Experimental Research, 4*(2), 135–145.

Spohr, H.L., & Steinhausen, H.C. (1984). A retrospective four-year follow-up study of children with the Fetal Alcohol Syndrome: Clinical psychopathological and development aspects. In M. O'Connor & J. Whelan (Eds.), *Mechanisms of alcohol damage in utero*, CIBA Foundation Symposium No. 105 (pp. 197–217). London: Pitman.

Steinhausen, H.C., Nestler, V., & Spohr, H.L. (1982). Development and psychopathology of children with the fetal alcohol syndrome. *Developmental and Behavioral Pediatrics, 3*(2), 49–54.

Streissguth, A.P. (1986a). The behavioral teratology of alcohol: Performance, behavioral, and intellectual deficits in prenatally exposed children (pp. 3–44). In J.R. West (Ed.), *Alcohol and brain development*. New York: Oxford University Press.

Streissguth, A.P. (1986b). Smoking and drinking during pregnancy and offspring learning disabilities. In M. Lewis (Ed.), *Learning disabilities and prenatal risk* (pp. 28–67). Urbana-Champaign, Illinois: University of Illinois Press.

Streissguth, A.P., Clarren, S.K., & Jones, K.L. (1985). Natural history of the Fetal Alcohol Syndrome: A ten-year follow-up of eleven patients. *Lancet, II*, 85–92.

Streissguth, A.P., Herman, C.S., & Smith, D.W. (1978a). Intelligence, behavior and dysmorphogenesis in the Fetal Alcohol Syndrome: A report on 20 patients. *Journal of Pediatrics, 92*(3), 363–367.

Streissguth, A.P., Herman, C.S., Smith, D.W. (1978b). Stability of intelligence in the fetal alcohol syndrome: A preliminary report. *Alcoholism: Clinical and Experimental Research,* 2(2), 165–170.

Streissguth, A.P., Landesman-Dwyer, S., Martin, J.C., & Smith, D.W. (1980). Teratogenic effects of alcohol in humans and laboratory animals. *Science, 209*, 353–361.

Streissguth, A.P., & Martin, J.C. (1983). Prenatal effects of alcohol abuse in humans and laboratory animals. In B. Kissin, & H. Begleiter (Eds.), *The pathogenesis of alcoholism*, (Vol. 7, pp. 539–589). New York: Plenum Press.

Stromland, K. (1985). Ocular abnormalities in the fetal alcohol syndrome. *Acta Opthamologica*, Supplement 171, 63.

Sullivan, W.C. (1899). A note on the influence of maternal inebriety on the offspring. *Journal of Mental Science, 45*, 489–503.

Surgeon General's Advisory on Alcohol and Pregnancy. (1981). *FDA Drug Bulletin*, 11(2).

Taylor, A.N., Nelson, L.R., Branch, B.J., Kokka, N., & Poland, R.E. (1984). Altered stress responsiveness in adult rats exposed to ethanol in utero: Neuroendocrine mechanisms. In M. O'Connor & J. Whelan (Eds.), CIBA Foundation Symposium No. 105: *Mechanisms of Alcohol Damage in Utero*. London: Pitman.

Van Thiel, D.H., Parker, S., Udani, M., & Gavaler, J.S. (1984). Adverse effects of ethanol on the adult sexual behavior of male rats exposed in utero. *Neurobehavioral Toxicology and Teratology, 6,* 289–293.

Vorhees, C.V. (1986). Principles of behavioral teratology. In E.P. Riley & C.V. Vorhees (Eds.), *Handbook of behavioral teratology*. New York: Plenum Press.

Warner, R.H., & Rosett, H.L. (1975). The effects of drinking on offspring: An historical survey of the American and British literature. *Journal of Studies on Alcohol, 36*(11), 1395–1420.

West, J.R. (1986). *Alcohol and brain development*. New York: Oxford University Press.

Wilson, J.G. (1977). Current status of teratology. In J.G. Wilson & F.C. Fraser (Eds.), *Handbook of teratology: Vol. 1. General principles and etiology* (pp. 47–74). New York: Plenum Press.

Fetal Antigenicity and Maternal Immunoreactivity Factors in Mental Retardation

C. Thomas Gualtieri
University of North Carolina

The known causes of mental retardation account for only a small minority of cases. There remains an "unexplained residue . . . of staggering proportions" (Medawar, 1963).

The uterine environment of the human fetus is increasingly called to attention as a likely candidate to reduce this "unexplained residue." Here the developing organism is most vulnerable to environmental influences: to viruses and other infectious agents, to endocrine and nutritional effects, and to the consequences of the maternal immunologic response. The antenatal environment of the human fetus plays a signal role in the development of the person. The antigenic nature of the fetus and the immunoreactive idiosyncrasies of his/her mother play a central role in determining what that environment will be.

> "The concurrent evolution of viviparity and the ability to render an immunologic response to foreign antigens raised certain problems for the fetus." (Medawar, 1963, p. 324)
>
> "Pregnancy is associated with the development of circulating maternal antibodies directed against the histocompatability antigens of the fetus simultaneously with the specific inhibition of immune reactivity against the fetus as a graft." (Simmons, 1971, p. 407)

The mechanisms by which the fetus is protected against the circulating antibodies and effector lymphocytes of the mother have been of considerable interest to transplantation biologists, oncologists, and other scientists; the topic has been reviewed on several occasions (Bernard, 1977; Billingham, 1964; Simmons, 1971). The mechanisms by which the

Acknowledgement. The authors wish to acknowledge the contributions the following persons made to the preparation of this manuscript: Susan Council, La Sharon Lee, Morris Lipton, James Mayo, and Debra Patterson. Work was supported in part by grants from the National Institute of Child Health and Human Development (HD 07201) and from the National Institute of Mental Health (MH 33127).

fetus as an allograft is protected from maternal immune attack are still imperfectly understood (Simmons, 1971), but it is known that fetal immunoprotection is not perfect. Fetal antigens and cells can enter the maternal circulation and maternal antibodies and (possibly) effector lymphocytes enter the fetal circulation (Adinolfi, 1976; Adinolfi, Beck, Haddad, & Seller, 1976; Barnes & Tuffrey, 1971). A cell-mediated immune response can develop in mothers during pregnancy. It may increase in intensity with gestation and increase even more so with succeeding pregnancies (Burke & Johansen, 1974; Doughty & Gelsthorpe, 1976; Johansen & Burke, 1974; Terasaki, Mickey, Yamazaki, & Vredevoe, 1970).

In response to fetal antigens of the human lymphocytotoxic antigen (HLA) class, maternal lymphocytotoxic antibody production increases with the first three or four pregnancies and then levels off (Doughty & Gelsthorpe, 1976). It has been hypothesized that if certain kinds of cytotoxic antibodies reach critical levels in the maternal circulation, they will exceed the number of available binding sites on the placenta and enter the fetal circulation (Doughty & Gelsthorpe, 1974). Other fetal antigens may also play a role in maternal immunoreactivity; for example, the blood group antigen (ABO) system may also contribute to maternal immune sensitivity, and ABO incompatibility between mother and fetus is known to contribute to increased fetal wastage (Cohen & Mellitts, 1971). In the author's analysis of data from the British Perinatal Study (Butler & Bonham, 1963), it was discovered that perinatal mortality increased more sharply with parity in O-type mothers, who are more likely to react to fetal red blood cell antigens, than in A, B, or AB mothers. (Gualtieri & Hicks, 1985a)

There seems to be substantial interindividual variation in the maternal immune response (Lawler, Ukaejoofo, & Reeves, 1975). In one study, only 15% of pregnancies were characterized by the development of maternal HLA antibodies (Doughty & Gelsthorpe, 1974). Medawar has shown that antigenic incompatibility is a necessary but not a sufficient cause for Rh disease (Loke, 1978; Medawar, 1963); isoimmunization is necessary, but not sufficient, to produce hemolytic anemia in the newborn (Medawar, 1963). In fact, there is a wide range of reactivity between maternal and fetal lymphocytes (Lawler et al., 1975).

Fetal immunoprotection seems to be less perfect for the male fetus, and this may be the consequence of the sex-linked antigen H-Y, probably acting in concert with other antigen systems. Sex differences in antigenicity were first described in the *Eichwald-Silmser effect:* male skin grafts survive less well in female animals than do male-to-male, female-to-male, or female-to-female allografts (Eichwald & Silmser, 1955). Trophoblast grafts from female concepti survive longer than male trophoblasts (Borland, Loke, & Oldersnaw, 1970); most choriocarcinomas arise from female concepti (Scott, 1976) and those which arise from male concepti are notably less aggressive (Loke, 1978).

There is clinical evidence that male fetuses are more antigenic than females: immune complexes are found more frequently in the cord blood of male newborns (Farber, Cambiaso, & Masson, 1981); runt disease and Rh disease occur more commonly in males (Beer & Billingham, 1973; Scott & Beer, 1973); toxemia, which is probably an autoimmune disorder, is more common when the fetus is male and the sex ratio increases proportionately with the severity of the disease (Toivanen & Hirvonen, 1970b).

The identification of a male-specific antigen termed H-Y was originally made in connection with the Eichwald-Silmser effect (*vide infra*) (Ohno, 1979). The expression of H-Y antigen probably derives from a monomorphic gene locus (Ohno, 1979). The original hypothesis was that H-Y antigen is specified by a gene located on the Y chromosome (Goodfellow & Andrews, 1982), but Wolf (1981) has presented evidence to suggest that the structural gene for H-Y antigen is autosomal and that its expression is regulated by an X-linked repressor and a Y-linked inducer.

Whatever the genetic origin of H-Y antigen, there is no disagreement over issues of ubiquity or specificity. H-Y antigen has been shown to be conserved to the extreme throughout vertebrate evolution (Ohno, 1979). Having performed an extensive series of H-Y antibody absorption tests, Wachtel, Koo, & Boyse (1975) demonstrated that male cells of all mammalian species tested, including man, absorbed out the male-specific cytotoxicity of H-Y antibody, while no crossreacting materials were found on female cells (Ohno, 1979). H-Y antigen is ubiquitously expressed in every somatic cell type of the mammalian male (Ohno, 1979). It is first expressed in pre-implantation male embryos at the eight-cell stage (Krco & Goldberg, 1976). An exact and invariant function seems to have been assigned by evolution to H-Y antigen and, as far as mammals are concerned, it is felt to lie in the determination of primary (gonadal) sex; H-Y is an absolute prerequisite, though it is not necessarily sufficient, for testicular organization (Ohno, 1979).

Although H-Y is the prime candidate to account for the hypothesized antigenicity of the male fetus, it is a minor histocompatibility antigen, a weak immunogen, and its effects may be exercised in clinically important ways only through a cumulative effect with other antigens, including those of the ABO (Toivanen & Hirvonen, 1970a), Rh (Scott & Beer, 1973; Renkonen & Timonen, 1967) or HLA systems (Goulmy, Termijtelen, Bradley, & Van Rood, 1977; Johansen, Festenstein, & Burke, 1974; Loke, 1978). Alternatively, maternal-fetal immunoreactivity could be mediated in males whose mothers are sensitized to other antigens but not to H-Y or in females, who do not express H-Y antigen by virtue of an X-linked antigenic system (e.g., H-X, Xg[a]) (Berryman & Silvers, 1979; Loke, 1978) that may have clinical importance.

There are known pathologic consequences of maternal immune attack on the fetus—for example, Rh disease and runt disease, as mentioned above. ABO incompatibility between mother and fetus is associated with an increased perinatal mortality (Cohen & Mellitts, 1971). Other examples include autoimmune thrombocytopenia and autoimmune hemolytic anemia, myasthenia gravis, thyroiditis, and the lupus erythematosis (LE) phenomenon and cardiomyopathy in children of mothers with systemic lupus erythematosis (SLE) (Beer & Billingham, 1973; Brent, 1971; Bresnihan, Grigor, Oliver, Leiskomia, & Hughes, 1977; Kitzmiller, 1978). In the latter condition, there is known to be transplacental transfer of antinuclear antibody from mother to fetus (Beck & Rowell, 1963).

Autoimmune disorders are good examples of how maternal immunoreactivity can afflict the fetus. Some autoimmune disorders, such as rheumatoid arthritis, tend to remit during pregnancy, while others, such as SLE, often arise during pregnancy (Bresnihan et al., 1977; Kitzmiller, 1978). In autoimmune hemolytic anemia, the disorder may remit postpartum, only to arise again with a subsequent pregnancy (Kitzmiller, 1978). Increased fetal loss through spontaneous abortion is seen in SLE, schleroderma, autoimmune hemolytic anemia, and autoimmune thrombocytopenic purpura (Kitzmiller, 1978). Fetal wastage is increased in SLE mothers even before the disease is clinically manifest (Kitzmiller, 1978). Lymphocytotoxic antibody titres are higher in SLE mothers who had spontaneous abortions than in mothers who had normal live births (Bresnihan et al., 1977). Toxemia is more common in mothers with SLE (Kitzmiller, 1978). And, based on the present author's review of an admittedly sparse literature, more girls than boys are born to mothers with SLE.

In a study of women who gave birth to children with congenital heart block, a significant association was found between the occurrence of the disease and the transplacental passage of anti-Ro (SS-A) antibody from the mother to the baby (Scott et al., 1983). This antibody is also associated with other types of pregnancy pathology. It is directly toxic in various tissue culture systems and is reactive with heart and brain cells under certain conditions (Taylor, 1985). It is of further interest that Ro (SS-A) antigen has been shown to be ten times more abundant in heart and brain than in any other body tissues (Wolin & Steitz, 1984).

The brain may be an immunologically privileged site in some respects, but immune attack on nervous tissue does occur in conditions like multiple sclerosis, polyneuropathy, and spongiform encephalopathy (Abramsky, Lisalc, Silberger, & Pleasure, 1977; Dalakas & Engel, 1981; Hauser et al., 1983; Sotelo, Gibbs, & Gadjusek, 1980). Neurobiologists continue to pursue the possibility of autoimmune mechanisms in the genesis of some forms of schizophrenia (Abramsky and Litvin, 1978; McPherson, 1970).

Brain tissue is antigenic (Foster & Archer, 1979). It shares antigens with other tissues including histocompatibility antigens, organ specific antigens, and antigens present on tissue cells (Foster & Archer, 1979; Roszkowski, Plaut, & Lichtenstein, 1977). There are brain antigens specific to neurons and oligodendroglia (Poduslo, McFarland, & McKahanon, 1977); there are antigens specific to cells in functional groups (Williams & Schupf, 1977) or anatomic areas (Blessing, Costa, Gefen, & Rush, 1977); there are antigens specific to subcellular components of neural tissue (Sotelo et al., 1980). Antibodies to brain antigens can act as teratogens when injected into pregnant animals (Brent, 1971). Rats and guinea pigs immunized to nerve growth factor (NGF) develop anti-NGF antibodies that attack fetal nervous tissue *in utero* when the animals are bred (Johnson, Gorin, Brandeis, & Pearson, 1980). The immature blood-brain barrier is not capable of protecting the developing brain from damage by maternal antibodies or effector lymphocytes (Adinolfi, 1976; Adinolfi et al., 1976).

It is not the present author's purpose to review vast research areas having to do with the immunoprotection of pregnancy or the immunopathology of brain. Nor can the precise immunopathic mechanisms be described that mediate maternal attack and induce neuropathic changes in the fetus. Nor can one specify whether H-Y antigen alone is involved, or whether there are other important antigens in the male at particular points in time during gestation, or whether incompatibility in other antigen systems, like HLA and ABO, may also play a role and, if so, whether the reaction that ensues is additive or multiplicative. These are grounds for speculation and basic research. Sufficient to guide this argument are the following conclusions, which are fair and conservative: fetal immunoprotection is not invariant or complete; breakdowns in the system do occur, with occasional pathologic consequences to the fetus, occurring along a continuum of severity; the brain, especially the fetal brain, is not invulnerable to immune attack; and in laboratory animals at least, maternal antibodies can damage the developing nervous tissue of the fetus.

The idea that male antigenicity or maternal immunoreactivity may exert a negative influence on the neurological development of children has been suggested on previous occasions by Adinolfi (1976), Loke (1978), Foster and Archer (1979), Rubenstein (1982), and Singer, Westphal and Niswander (1968). The hypothesis has usually been advanced on the basis of indirect evidence, for example, to explain the prevalence of pregnancy complications in males (Singer et al., 1968) or the negative parity effect on

IQ (Foster & Archer, 1979). Adinolfi based his argument on the immaturity of the fetal blood-brain barrier (Adinolfi et al., 1976), the detection of maternal specific antibodies in the CSF of infants tested during the first week of life (Thorley, Holmes, Kaplan, McCracken, & Sanford, 1975), and supporting data from preclinical experiments (Adinolfi, 1976). There is additional direct evidence, but not much.

In 1978, Bonner et al. reported cytotoxic antibodies in the sera of 574 parous women (Bonner et al., 1978); 25% had cytotoxins after their first pregnancy and 50% after the sixth. Children with congenital anomalies were more likely to be born to mothers who developed cytotoxic antibodies. Harris and London (1976) reported that mothers with lymphocytotoxic antibodies were more likely to show signs of maternal insufficiency (pre-eclampsia, fetal distress, carbohydrate intolerance, unexplained fetal death, intrauterine growth retardation, congenital anomaly, and premature labor) than mothers with no lymphocytotoxic antibodies. In a group of twenty women with repeated miscarriage, Bardawil, Mitchell, McKeogh, and Marchant (1962) reported that they manifested rapid rejection of skin grafts from husbands four times more frequently than grafts that were made from unrelated donors (Loke, 1978). In a mixed lymphocyte reaction paradigm, the percentage of transformed cells was discovered to be lower in normal fertile couples and higher in infertile couples; a dosage effect was observed in women who had had repeated miscarriage (Halbrecht & Komlos, 1976; Ohama & Kadotani, 1971). Finally, in two papers from the Soviet Union, it was reported that mothers with "antibrain antibodies" were more likely to give birth to children with developmental or neurological disorders (Burbaeva, 1972; Kolyaskina, Boehme, Buravlev, & Faktor, 1977).

It becomes increasingly apparent that the immunologic environment of the fetus and occasional imperfections in the system of fetal immunoprotection represent important new areas to pursue in order to establish new causes of mental retardation and severe mental illness. Because fetal antigenicity is compounded in the male by the presence of H-Y antigen, maternal-fetal immunoreactivity becomes an important candidate to explain the phenomenon of selective male affliction with these conditions.

SELECTIVE MALE AFFLICTION

Males are selectively afflicted with virtually every neurologic, psychiatric, and developmental disorder of childhood (see Table 1). There are notable conditions, of course, like anencephaly and dysraphism, that are more common in females (Glucksmann, 1978; Nakano, 1973); but for the most important neurodevelopmental disorders—mental retardation,

TABLE 1

Male-Female Differences in Developmental Neuropsychiatry and Obstetrics

DISORDER	SEX RATIO[a]	REFERENCE(S)
A. PEDIATRIC PSYCHIATRY		
Hyperkinetic syndrome	300	(Butler & Bonham, 1963; Trites, Dugas, Lynch, & Gerguson, 1979)
Conduct disorders	270	(Rutter, 1970; Trites et al., 1979)
	200–900	(Zerssen & Weyerer, 1982)
Childhood schizophrenia	170	(Kramer, 1978)
Early onset schizophrenia	160	(Samuels, 1979; Flor-Henry, 1974)
Process schizophrenia	150	(Flor-Henry, 1974; Allon, 1971)
Suicide		(Shaffer & Fisher, 1981)
Referrals to child psychiatry clinics	200	(Taylor & Ounsted, 1972)
Admission to child psychiatric service	213	(Gualtieri, 1983)
B. PEDIATRIC NEUROLOGY		
Seizure disorders		
All ages	120	(Taylor & Ounsted, 1972)
Neonatal convulsions	116	(Taylor & Ounsted, 1972)
Childhood seizures	140	(Taylor & Ounsted, 1972)
Infantile spasms	210	(Taylor & Ounsted, 1972)
Temporal lobe epilepsy	132	(Taylor & Ounsted, 1972)
Febrile seizures	140	(Taylor & Ounsted, 1972)
In mentally retarded children	170	(Corbett et al., 1975)
Cerebral palsy	150–260	(Wing, 1981; Taylor & Ounsted, 1972)
SSPE	220	(Taylor & Ounsted, 1972)
Encephalitis (Echo Type 9)	220	(Sabin et al., 1958)
Abnormal neurological exam at 1 year of age	114	(Singer et al., 1968)
C. DEVELOPMENTAL DISORDERS		
Severe mental retardation	130	(Abramowicz & Richardson, 1975)
Down syndrome	128–260	(Tsai & Beisler, 1983; Burgio, Fraccaro, Ticpolo, & Wolf, 1981)
Speech and language disorders	260	(Ingram, 1959)
Stuttering	400	(Reinisch et al., 1979)
Learning difficulties	219	(Nichols & Chen, 1981)
Dyslexia	430	(McKinney & Feagans, 1983)
Autism	400	(Ingram, 1964)
D. OBSTETRICS/PERINATAL		
Spontaneous abortion	120–140	(McMillen, 1979)
Toxemia	109–171	(Toivanen & Hirvonen, 1970)
Placenta praevia	120	(Ounsted, 1972)
Abruptio placentae	206	(Ounsted, 1972)
Antepartum hemorrhage	140–210	(Rhodes, 1965)
Intrapartum anoxia	130	(Butler & Bonham, 1963)
Pulmonary infection	250	(Butler & Bonham, 1963)
Hyaline membrane disease	180	(Butler & Bonham, 1963)
Pulmonary hemorrhage	210	(Butler & Bonham, 1963)
Cerebral birth trauma	180	(Butler & Bonham, 1963)
Apgar 6	130	(Singer et al., 1968)

[a]The sex ratio is expressed, by convention, as the number of males divided by the number of females multiplied by one hundred, or $(N^m/N^f)100$.

autism, hyperactivity, dyslexia, epilepsy, dysphasia, cerebral palsy, and conduct disorders—the sex differential works unequivocally to male disadvantage (Butler & Bonham, 1963; Nichols & Chen, 1981; Rutter, 1970). This biological prejudice is largely unexplained.

It has been suggested that the genetic endowment of the male comprises sufficient cause for male "inferiority" (Childs, 1965; Ounsted & Taylor, 1972; Rutter, 1970). The Y chromosome is considerably smaller than the X is, and also "curiously inert," thus giving the female a "4–5% quantitative superiority in genetic material" (Childs, 1965). This disparity means that the homogametic sex (females) must always be haploid. Because there are loci on the X chromosome that control functions apart from reproductive sex, males are necessarily the victims of whatever "uncompensated dosage effects" may exist (Childs, 1965). X linkage has been proposed to account for greater male variability in virtually all biological traits, including mental functioning (Lehrke, 1978). Untoward X-linked recessive genes are expressed in males but not in heterozygous females, and the occurrence of X-linked disorders of development is not infrequent. However, such occurrences are not sufficiently frequent to account for the breadth and ubiquity of the phenomenon of selective affliction. Most of the conditions in Table 1 are not X linked and the large majority do not show the pattern of inheritance that characterizes specific chromosomal abnormalities.

The effect of the Y chromosome message has been described by Ounsted and Taylor (1972) as *catalytic;* that is, it serves to "modify any genome." Females express neither the fullest advantages nor the worst disadvantages of their genome. Their characteristics are said to be "less scattered," while males suffer the "extremes of viable disadvantage and the greatest advantage" (Ounsted & Taylor, 1972). Thus male inferiority is said to be the consequence of greater genetic variability for "the majority of measurable characteristics" (Wing, 1981).

According to the hypothesis of Ounsted and Taylor, the increased variability expressed in males is at least in part a consequence of the function of the Y chromosome in regulating the pace of development. "Transcription of expressed genomic information in males occurs at a slower developmental pace; the operation of the Y chromosome is to allow more genomic information to be transcribed" (Ounsted & Taylor, 1972). Whether or not the pace of development is regulated by the Y chromosome—and there is, to the present author's knowledge, no direct evidence that it is—it is an incontestable fact that development and maturation occurs more slowly in males (D. Taylor, 1969). At every developmental stage, the male is less mature than the female (D. Taylor, 1969). A newborn girl is the physiological equivalent of a 4- to 6-week-old boy (Hutt, 1972). In general, immature organisms are more susceptible to damage than mature ones (Rutter, 1970) and the developing male is more susceptible "to the information he extracts from his genome and the environment" (Taylor & Ounsted, 1972). Thus, relative immaturity means that males are more vulnerable to environmental factors for a longer period of time; these factors may be intrauterine, peri- or postnatal, psychosocial or biologic. The classic and often cited example of the untoward clinical sequellae of prolonged immaturity was put forth by Taylor and Ounsted (1971). The interval of susceptibility to convulsive seizures originating in the temporal lobe as a consequence of cerebral injury is considerably longer in the male infant.

The complement to prolonged maturation is increased complexity; the male human is said to be a more complex organism than the female and his brain is a more complex organ. The male brain is more "completely" lateralized (McGlone, 1980), it is heavier (Dekaban & Sadowsky, 1978), its oxygen requirements are higher (Hutt, 1972), it is an "androgenized" female brain (Reinisch, Gandelman, & Spiegel, 1979). If male brain development is more complicated and prolonged, "there are likely to be more opportunities for errors to occur" (Reinisch et al., 1979). However, this theory is not explicit as to how, precisely, these errors come about, or what, precisely, they are, at least on a physiologic basis. By the same token, the immaturity hypothesis fails to describe any specifics about the information the developing child "extracts" from his genome or his environment, or how this process unfolds.

Male vulnerability is, of course, hardly limited to congenital disorders, and no review of the topic can afford to overlook the general pattern of male vulnerability, at every age, to accident and disease. (The notable exceptions are the autoimmune diseases and, of course, diseases of the female reproductive organs (Rutter, 1970; Vessey, 1972)). The higher mortality of males is reflected in the sex ratio ((male:females) x 100). Although the primary sex ratio (i.e., at conception) is probably around 120 (estimated range 110–170) (McMillen, 1979), male fetuses are more prone to spontaneous abortion and stillbirth (McMillen, 1979), and by the end of gestation the (secondary) sex ratio falls to about 105. By the end of childhood, the sex ratio drops to unity, a consequence of increased male mortality from accidents and childhood diseases (Reinisch et al., 1979).

It is not likely, however, that this general and lifelong pattern of male vulnerability can be molded to accommodate a single, parsimonious, and unifying theory, or at least one that would make sense or generate testable hypotheses. The range of problems to which males succumb is simply too broad; each is probably the consequence of a host of different intervening variables. The specific area of concern here, the neurodevelopmental disorders of childhood, also comprises a broad and diverse range of problems, but this topic is more tractable and one that may well be open to intelligent theory.

It is a fair surmise that most of the foregoing ideas about selective male affliction may succeed as explanations or as seminal ideas, but that they fail as theories; their capacity to generate testable hypotheses seems to be extremely limited. It is concluded, with Butler, that "the explanation for most of these striking [sex] differences is not understood" (Butler & Bonham, 1963).

THE STRUCTURE OF SEX DIFFERENCES

"In general, the morbific processes, mild and grave, attack the females with greater intensity than the males" (Ciocco, 1940).

While females are less liable to affliction with neurodevelopmental problems, when such conditions do arise in the female, a severer form is usually manifest (Taylor & Ounsted, 1972). This principle seems to hold for most of the pathologic conditions in which it has been tested. For example, although males are more frequently found to be mentally retarded, at the lowest levels of IQ the proportion of females is relatively higher (Taylor & Ounsted, 1972). Autistic children are more commonly males, but at the lowest IQ levels the number of autistic females is proportionately higher (Lord, Schopler, & Revicki, 1982; Lotter, 1974; Tsai & Beisler, 1983; Tsai, Stewart, & August, 1981; Wing, 1981). The mortality rate of people who are retarded and institutionalized (Forssman & Akesson, 1970) and of Downs children (Fabia & Drolette, 1970) is higher in females and the mortality rate of females with cerebral palsy is also higher (Ingram, 1964; Schlesinger, Alaway & Peltin, 1959). Females are less prone to epilepsy, but they are more prone to the morbid sequellae of febrile seizures (Taylor & Ounstead, 1972) and to the development of epileptic psychosis (Flor-Henry, 1969; M. Taylor, 1969; Slater, Beard, & Glithero, 1963; Taylor & Ounsted, 1972). In order to understand why this is an important point, it is essential to consider the structure of male-female differences as they relate to the disorders in question, and especially as they relate to the occurrence of perinatal problems.

In the neurodevelopmental disorders, sex differences confer a dissociation between the elements of frequency (or incidence) and intensity (or severity). As a general rule, males are more frequently afflicted and females more severely impaired when they are afflicted. Additional sex-based dissociations are that the occurrence of neurodevelopmental disorders in females seems to be mediated primarily through genetic channels and that their disorders may be, as a consequence, more specific, while in males, the disorders are mediated largely through the occurrence of perinatal problems and are less specific and more diverse in their manifestation. There is strong suggestive evidence for this.

The occurrence of "pure-type" dyslexia is more frequent in girls (Pennington & Smith, 1983) and it is possible to fit a genetic model to learning disabilities in girls but not in boys (Lewitter, DeFries, & Elston, 1980). The clinical picture of autistic children with positive family histories of developmental dysfunction is more homogeneous than for those with negative family histories (August, Stewart, & Tsai, 1981). The range of IQ in autistic males is wider (Wing, 1981). Autistic girls are more likely than boys to have family histories of cognitive and language dysfunction (Tsai & Beisler, 1983) and members of the families of dyslexic girls (Decker & DeFries, 1980) and of girls with conduct disorders (Robins, 1966) are more frequently afflicted. The clinical presentation of a disorder that is largely mediated by the genotype is likely to be more specific, while the behavioral and developmental sequellae of early brain damage are known to be relatively nonspecific (Graham & Rutter, 1968).

The same pattern is suggested by studies of the genetics of schizophrenia. For example, the concordance for schizophrenia in MZ twins is higher for females than males (Rosenthal, 1962). Schizophrenic mothers of children who become schizophrenic tend themselves to have had an earlier onset of the disorder (Mednick, 1970) and the births of such children are characterized by relative difficulty (Mednick, 1970; Mednick, Mura, Schulsinger, & Mednick, 1971). However, severity of the maternal illness is associated with the level of schizophrenia only in high risk daughters and not in sons (Gardner, 1967; Sobel, 1961); perinatal complications, on the other hand, are more likely in high risk sons and less in daughters (Mednick, Schulsinger, Teasdale, Schulsinger, Venables, & Rock, 1977). There is a significant relationship between perinatal complications and the later development of schizophrenia in high risk boys but not in girls (Mednick et al., 1977). The daughters of schizophrenic mothers are likely to be schizophrenic if they have any disorder at all, while the sons exhibit a more diverse range of psychopathology, especially sociopathy and criminal behavior. What this suggests is that "schizophrenia in females is more genetically determined and that schizophrenia in males has a heavier environmental weight" (Mednick et al., 1977). When the high risk daughters of schizophrenic mothers develop schizophrenia, it is largely (though not entirely) determined by their genotype; the sons develop schizophrenia or other severe psychiatric disorders, and this is mediated by a genotype by environment interaction. The environmental effect is keenly felt by males during pregnancy and parturition.

Schizophrenia is not properly counted among the neurodevelopmental disorders (although a cogent case might be made that it should be), especially the form of schizophrenia with early onset, which occurs more commonly in males, responds poorly to treatment, is often associated with demonstrable neuropathic changes, and follows a dementing course (Weinberger, Cannon-Spoor, Potkin, & Wyatt, 1980).

The author observed a similar structure in the sex differences in developmentally handicapped children. In a retrospective review of 223 developmentally handicapped children referred for evaluation at the University of North Carolina within a given year, the majority were, as expected, male (78%). In terms of IQ and SQ (social quotient), however, the females were more severely impaired (Table 2, A). For both males and females, there was a positive linear relationship between the occurrence of newborn problems (e.g., hypoxia, jaundice) and IQ (F^{Linear} (1,166) = 5.255, p = .025) and SQ (F^{Linear} (1,185) = 4.715, p = .025), and between

TABLE 2

The Structure of Sex Differences (Gualtieri & Hicks, 1985c)

A. Females are more severely impaired than males

		Males	Females
IQ	Mean	55.3	41.2
	S.D.	±23.7	±21.5
	N	139	35
	F (1,172) = 10.18, p = .002		

		Males	Females
SQ	Mean	63.0	52.9
	S.D.	±24.2	±18.9
	N	154	40
	F (1,192) = 6.0, p = .015		

B. Proportion of each sex classified by number of problems in pregnancy

	Pregnancy Problems			
	None	One	More than one	N
Boys	0.058	0.234	0.708	171
Girls	0.283	0.130	0.587	46
				217

Pearson $\chi^2 = 19.785$, p = .0001

C. Proportion of each sex classified by family history of neurodevelopmental disorders

	Relatives Affected	Relatives Not Affected	
Male Proband	21	146	167
Female Proband	11	31	42
	32	177	209

Pearson $\chi^2 = 4.798$, p = .05

the occurrence of neurological problems in the first year of life (e.g., seizures, dystonia) and IQ (F^{Linear} (1,168) = 11.907, p = .001) and SQ (F^{Linear} (1.188) = 10.713, p = .001). Newborn problems and first-year neurological problems were associated (Pearson χ^2 = 24.295, p = .0001). There was a positive relationship between newborn problems and low birthweight (F^{Linear} (1,204) = 8.087, p = .005) as well as with delivery complications (Pearson χ^2 = 21.7, p = .0002). Both newborn problems (F^{Linear} (1.172) = 8.521, p = .01) and neurological problems were associated with pregnancy complications (F^{Linear} (1,174) = 15.147, p = .001). However, pregnancy complications were significantly more common in males (Table 2, B). On the other hand, a family history of neurodevelopmental disorders was more frequent in females (Table 2, C). The severity of affliction was worse for females and their genetic background was less decisive (Hicks & Gualtieri, 1985).

Sex differences occurring in the neurodevelopmental disorders of childhood contain four elements: males are more commonly afflicted; when females *are* afflicted, the manifestation of the condition is more severe; in females, such disorders are largely influenced by the genotype and as a consequence, the manifestation is more specific; in males, the occurrence of neurodevelopmental disorders is mediated by a genotype by environment interaction, pre- and perinatal problems play a more important role and the manifestation is more diverse.

Such a pattern is consistent with a model that posits a spectrum or a continuum of liability. Liability to a neurodevelopmental disorder is a function of a number of genes acting in concert; these polygenes are presumed to be normally distributed within the population. The essential part of this model is a differential threshold for expression of the phenotype for males and females. For females, a substantial genetic load is required. This threshold of liability model was originally proposed by Carter to account for sex differences in the occurrence of certain congenital malformations (1965) and the model has also been advanced with respect to dyslexia (Lewitter, DeFries, & Elston, 1980), conduct disorder and sociopathy (Cloninger, Christiansen, Reich, & Gottesman, 1978), stuttering (Garside & Kay, 1964), left handedness (Hicks & Kinsbourne, 1981), autism (Tsai & Beisler, 1983), pyloric stenosis (Carter, 1965) and cleft lip and palate (Woolf, 1971).

It is suggested that the threshold for expression of neurodevelopmental problems in males is lower by virtue of their proclivity to encounter serious and damaging pre- and perinatal difficulties. It is not necessary to postulate an increased level of *vulnerability* to such difficulties for males, although this may be the case, simply because the very occurrence of pregnancy complications in males is substantially more frequent (Butler & Bonham, 1963; Nichols & Chen, 1981; Singer et al., 1968). The male fetus is much more likely to encounter intrauterine difficulties such as toxemia (Toivanen & Hirvonen, 1970b), abruptio placentae (Rhodes, 1965), placenta praevia (Ounsted, 1972), prematurity (Niswander & Gordon, 1972) and miscarriage (McMillen, 1979). It is well known that severe pre- and perinatal problems may cause or aggravate developmental problems and that less severe gestational events such as occasional bleeding are significantly associated with subsequent neurological, behavioral, and developmental problems (Nichols & Chen, 1981). The increased frequency with which males encounter an inhospitable uterine environment or a difficult passage compromises brain development and lowers their threshold of liability to neurodevelopmental problems.

The natural question here is why males are more prone to pre- and perinatal difficulties. Males are heavier *in utero* and at birth (Butler & Bonham, 1963) and larger fetuses are more prone to certain kinds of obstetrical and perinatal problems; but when birth weight is controlled, such problems are still more common in males (Singer et al., 1968). There seems to be something about the male fetus to evoke an untoward uterine environment.

MATERNAL INSUFFICIENCY AND NEGATIVE PARITY EFFECTS

Selective male affliction is hypothesized to arise as a consequence of a lowered threshold for expression of a deviant phenotype. The threshold is lowered through the mediation of complications of pregnancy and delivery. These occur more frequently in males, and "the female conceptus is better adapted to survive in the maternal uterine environment than the male" (Loke, 1978). An evocative principle is called for; what is it about the male fetus to cause such trouble? Fetal size is not a suitable candidate, but what may be?

There are two plausible alternatives: an endocrine effect or an antigenic effect. The former is a compelling idea because a male pregnancy is characterized by intermittent elevation of levels of testicular androgens (Mizuno, Lobotsky, Lloyd, Kobayashi, & Murasawa, 1968) and the balance among androgenic, progestational, and estrogenic hormones is known to affect fetal brain development (Maccoby, Doering, Jacklin, & Kraemer, 1979) and the gestational health of the mother (Siiteri, Febres, Clemens, Chang, Gondos, & Stites, 1977). The endocrine aspects of pregnancy and fetal brain development, however, are extraordinarily complex or even ambiguous, and the state of the science is not given in the author's opinion to a ready explanation of the phenomenon of selective affliction. In addition, data will be described immediately below that are probably incompatible with an endocrinologic viewpoint.

It is appropriate to explore two additional areas of study that have important bearing on the occurrence of perinatal complications: the issues of "maternal insufficiency" and the existence of parity effects in disorders of development. Together, they suggest that successive pregnancies are not independent events, that there exists a kind of memory in the phenomenon of reproduction—the fate of one pregnancy influences, or even predicts, the outcome of the next.

The term *maternal inadequacy* (Costeff, Cohen, Weller, & Kleckner, 1981) or *uterine inadequacy* (Ahern & Johnson, 1973) or *reduced optimality* (Gillberg & Gillberg, 1983) refers to the tendency of some mothers to experience an unusual degree of pre- and perinatal complications, including bleeding, toxemia, prematurity, difficult delivery, miscarriage, and perinatal death. As described above, the adequacy of a child's intrauterine environment exercises a substantial long term influence on his neurological and cognitive development (Joffe, 1969). "Maternal insufficiency" is an important risk factor in developmental disorders like autism (Aarkrog, 1968; Gillberg & Gillberg, 1983; Tsai & Beisler, 1983; Tsai et al., 1981), mental retardation, mild and severe (Costeff, Cohen, & Weller, 1983; Drillien, 1968; Hagberg, Hagberg, Lewerth, & Linberg, 1981; Lilienfield & Pasamanick, 1956), minimal brain dysfunction (MBD) (Gillberg & Rasmussen, 1982; Nichols & Chen, 1981), and childhood psychoses (Funderburk, Carter, Tanguay, Freeman, & Westlake, 1983), among others. There may be a dosage effect because signs of uterine inadequacy occur more frequently and in greater number in the more severe disorders such as autism than in MBD (Gillberg & Gillberg, 1983). It is also interesting that the signs of uterine inadequacy associated with certain disorders such as autism are not necessarily those that directly induce cerebral hypoxia (Gillberg & Gillberg, 1983).

Central to the concept of maternal insufficiency is the idea of a *tendency*. Although any mother can have an isolated bad pregnancy, there are some mothers who are unusually prone to bad pregnancies. This tendency is at least in part genetically determined; for example, the tendency to premature births is familial (Keller, 1981); there is a maternal genetic effect on the birth weight of cousins (Robson, 1955); and the aunts and sisters of mentally retarded children have more mental retardation, miscarriage, stillbirth, and neonatal death in their families than the uncles and brothers of mentally retarded children have in theirs (Ahern & Johnson, 1973). Daughters from toxemic pregnancies are affected themselves with toxemia more often than those from control groups (Chesley, Annito, & Cosgrove, 1968).

Because of familial uterine inadequacy, a troubled pregnancy does not occur as an independent event. The nature of one pregnancy is capable of predicting the nature of another. The birth weight of the first child is the most powerful predictor of low birth weight in the second (Bakketeig, 1977); the percentage of premature infants increases with the previous number of premature births (Placek, 1977); previous fetal or peri- or neonatal deaths predict similar deaths in subsequent pregnancies (Niswander & Gordon, 1972). And there is, again, an element of nonspecificity, as previous fetal loss predicts prematurity and previous prematurity predicts fetal loss (Niswander & Gordon, 1972; Placek, 1977). The first factor that operates here is the mother's constitutional insufficiency, which is genetic and probably speaks to a common underlying mechanism; the second factor is pre- or perinatal damage. The effects of this on the fetus are nonspecific.

A demonstration of how reproductive inefficiency of mothers of developmentally impaired children may be related to fetal antigenicity was provided by Costeff et al. (1981), who compared the incidence of complications of pregnancy, labor, and infancy in 87 mentally retarded children *(undifferentiated phenotype)* of consanguineous matings with 161 (idiopathic) mentally retarded children of nonconsanguineous matings. Complications were significantly more common in the latter group. Consanguineous matings, in which antigenic differences are minimized, were not associated with obstetrical or perinatal complications. The authors were led to speculate that "maternal (reproductive) inefficiency (i.e., obstetrical difficulties) may well reflect some so-far unidentified factor [which also causes] fetal brain damage" (Costeff et al., 1981).

Beyond the genetic memory of inherited inadequacy is another kind of memory that is expressed in the parity effect. *Parity effects* refer to systematic change in some measurable characteristic of offspring with increasing birth order or pregnancy order. Here again, there is a common pattern: the incidence of the complications of pregnancy and delivery, prematurity, miscarriage, and fetal and neonatal deaths increases with birth order; later born are at greater risk (Niswander & Gordon, 1972). Parity effects are also observed in at least some of the neurodevelopmental disorders, for example, mental retardation (Belmont, Stein, & Wittes, 1976), MBD (Badian, 1984; Nichols & Chen, 1981; Schrag, 1973), and autism (*vide infra*). A retarded, hyperactive, or learning disabled child is more frequently later born.

Maternal insufficiency has a predictable negative effect on pregnancies occurring within an extended family. The effects of maternal insufficiency seem to be mediated, however, within a sibship by the parity effect, with an increasingly negative impact on successive pregnancies. This incremental phenomenon is a form of nongenetic memory. It is consistent with the idea that some kind of sensitization process is at work. What could be inherited as maternal insufficiency is, in fact, a genetic proclivity to react immunologically to fetal antigen. The ensuing maternal immune attack against the fetus might seem to the clinician to be a complication of pregnancy and a sign of an inadequate uterine environment.

Selective male affliction, or at least a portion of it, is mediated through complications of pregnancy and childbirth, which occur more frequently in males. An evocative principle was postulated to characterize the male fetus and to render the occurrence of such complications more likely. The phenomenon of maternal insufficiency suggests a genetic element at play on the antigenic, but does not propose an endocrine explanation to the phenomenon on the fetal side. The evocative principle, therefore, is deduced to be the unique antigenic character of the male fetus.

Antigenic differences between zygote and mother are thought to confer an implantation advantage (Kirby, McWhirter, Teitelbaum, & Darlington, 1967). Trophoblastic invasion of the uterine decidua may be more extensive if the fetus is antigenically dissimilar to the mother, a mechanism that seems designed to promote genetic diversity (Brent, 1971). The male zygote, by virtue of its greater antigenic dissimilarity, is the beneficiary of this putative implantation advantage (Brent, 1971). Thus, the special antigenic character of the male fetus was first studied in connection with studies of the sex ratio. The secondary sex ratio, or sex ratio at birth, favors males in every human society that has been studied; the mean value for the United States is about 105 (Novitski, 1977). The primary sex ratio, that is, the sex ratio at conception, although difficult to measure, is even more favorable—around 120 (McMillen, 1979). As if to compensate for selective male affliction, nature has aspired to produce an excess of boys to begin with. The implantation advantage of antigenic dissimilarity has been proposed to account for this initial male advantage. Thus, the advantage enjoyed by males in the primary and secondary sex ratio has been attributed to their unique possession of H-Y antigen.

Sex differences in antigenicity may confer a growth advantage as well as an implantation advantage (Clarke & Kirby, 1966; Ounsted & Ounsted, 1970). Fetuses who are antigenically dissimilar to their mothers are likely to be larger (Clarke & Kirby, 1966) and the greater the antigenic dissimilarity, the greater the fetal growth rate (Ounsted & Ounsted, 1970). Male embryos, of course, grow faster than females: a baby boy is about 150 grams heavier than a girl at term. The sex ratio of large-for-dates infants is 150, while that of small-for-dates infants is 63 (Ounsted, 1972).

Placental weight is correlated with birth weight (Sedlis et al., 1967) and mammalian placentation also seems to be under some sort of immunologic control (Jones, 1968). In animal studies, antigenic dissimilarity is often found to promote placental growth (James, 1965). The placental size of male fetuses is larger (Ounsted, 1972); also interesting in light of the presumed autoimmune origin of the disorder is the fact that increased placental size is associated with the development of toxemia (Gleicher & Siegel, 1980). The sex ratio decreases with parity; with increasing birth order, fewer boys are born (Novitski & Sandler, 1956). An argument in favor of male antigenicity and maternal immunoreactivity has been raised to explain this phenomenon.

An antigenic explanation for the secondary sex ratio, implantation, placentation, and fetal growth suggests that maternal sensitization to male antigens occurs and affects subsequent pregnancies. The sex ratio decreases with parity, while birth weight and placental size increase (Niswander & Gordon, 1972; Novitski & Sandler, 1956; Vernier, 1975; Warburton & Naylor, 1971). The original implantation advantage enjoyed by the male zygote may be offset in subsequent pregnancies by the development of humoral antibodies or cell-mediated immune response in the mother. HLA antibodies, for example, develop in some mothers in response to pregnancy; with successive pregnancies, the number of HLA positive mothers increases (a ceiling seems to be reached at parity three or four) (Burke & Johansen, 1974; Doughty & Gelsthorpe, 1976). The sex ratio declines with parity in HLA positive mothers; in mothers who fail to develop HLA titres, the sex ratio actually increases with parity (Johansen & Burke, 1974). An early positive effect of immunoreactivity that serves to promote genetic diversity is balanced by a later negative effect, which seems to favor in large sibships the birth of the less expensive (female) sex.

If male fetuses are more antigenic, they should be more likely to sensitize mothers and the impact of this should be felt in subsequent pregnancies as changes in placentation and the sex ratio. In fact, predictions based on the antecedent brother effect seem to hold up. Placental size increases with parity in all-male sibships but not in all-female sibships; mixed sibships fall in between (Vernier, 1975). The sex ratio declines with parity if all of the antecedent siblings are male; it increases if antecedent siblings are all female (Gualtieri, Hicks, & Mayo, 1984; Renkonen, Makela, & Lehtovaara, 1962).

The parity effect on the sex ratio is mediated, it seems, through an *antecedent brother effect*. This effect has also been observed with respect to the occurrence of pregnancy complications in the past history of autistic children. The present author has reviewed the medical records of 209 autistic children who had been evaluated at the Medical School at the University of North Carolina. In 167 autistic boys, there was a significant relationship between the occurrence of pregnancy complications and the antecedent birth of brothers but not of sisters (see Table 3). Pregnancy complications were more common in autistic boys who had older brothers, but not in autistic boys who had older sisters. The number of autistic girls was too small to permit a complementary analysis.

TABLE 3

Antecedent Brother Effect on Complications of Pregnancy

167 Autistic Boys

		Antecedent Brothers		
		None	One	
Complications of pregnancy	None	12	2	14
	One	31	8	39
	More than one	71	43	114
		114	53	167

χ^2 for linear trend = 5.815, $p = .015$

		Antecedent Sisters		
		None	One	
Complications of pregnancy	None	8	6	14
	One	32	7	39
	More than one	79	35	114
		119	48	167

χ^2 for linear trend = 0.005, N.S.

The Immunoreactive Theory

Selective male affliction with the neurodevelopmental disorders may be related to male vulnerability to environmental stressors, to the genetic endowment of the male, or to his complexity and relative immaturity. In the author's opinion, these explanations are interesting but insufficient. They do not explain the male proclivity to encounter complications in pregnancy and childbirth. It is argued, with some support, that pregnancy complications mediate the occurrence of neurodevelopmental disorders more strongly in males than in females. The incidence of such complications in males leads to the postulation of an evocative principle, which may be hormonal or antigenic. The first alternative is attractive but inconsistent with the occurrence of parity effects in fetal loss and in at least some developmental disorders.

The antigenicity of the male fetus is consistent with the negative parity effect. The proposition that the male is especially antigenic and that some mothers are immunoreactors finds convincing support in the literature. The antigenicity of the male is probably related to the sex-linked H-Y antigen, although the immunogenicity of H-Y is probably enhanced and not diminished by it.

Maternal immune attack on the fetus is well known in a number of pathologic conditions and, when it occurs, it is the male who is more severely afflicted. Brain tissue is antigenic, the immature blood-brain barrier affords only slight protection from maternal immune attack, and maternal antibodies are sometimes found in the infant's cerebrospinal fluid (CSF). Congenital anomalies, infertility, and complications of pregnancy may occur in mothers with elevated antibody titres more frequently than in mothers with low or absent titres.

The argument is based on indirect evidence for the most part, although there is at least some direct supporting evidence. The relative paucity of direct support is not surprising. Although the theory of maternal-fetal immunoreactivity was first applied to studies of the sex ratio by Renkonen, Makela, and Lehtovaara in 1962, only a few scientists have even raised the question with respect to selective male affliction. Furthermore, the argument presented above relies heavily on the structure of sex differences in the occurrence of schizophrenia, and this dimorphic pattern has not been widely tested in clinical samples of developmentally handicapped children. When the present author did test the idea, it held up *(vide supra).* Finally, it is unfortunate when scientists who undertake studies of pregnancy complications and developmental disorders do not analyze their data by taking sex of the proband into consideration, but most do not.

The fundamental premise of the *Immunoreactive Theory* (IMRT) is that pregnancy is an immunological phenomenon characterized by a state of maternal tolerance. But fetal immunoprotection is relative, not absolute, and the system can break down. There is substantial interindividual variation in maternal-fetal immunoreactivity, but on the average male fetuses are more antigenic than females and maternal attack on the male embryo is more likely, especially if the mother's immunologic attack can be directed against fetal brain antigens.

Immunoreactivity is by no means put forth as a global explanation for all of the neuropathic disorders of childhood. The phenomenon may be robust but at the same time relatively weak and difficult to discern, especially in small clinical samples. Furthermore, the precise nature of the immunologic reaction cannot be described: whether it involves cell-mediated or humoral antibodies, whether a specific antigen, like H-Y, is responsible, or whether a number of fetal antigens or a combination thereof may be involved. Some fetal antigens may be short-lived and impossible to detect postnatally.

The author is aware that there is disagreement surrounding at least some of the "facts" upon which the theory is based. Parity estimates can be inaccurate, for example, as early investigators have agreed that placentation is promoted by antigenic similarity (Jones, 1968), or that the sex ratio decreases with antecedent brothers (McLaren, 1962), or that toxemia is an autoimmune disorder (Gleicher & Siegel, 1980). H-Y antigen is a fascinating new development in the study of sexual differentiation, but it is very difficult to measure (Goodfellow & Andrews, 1982). Nor is there any direct evidence that H-Y antigen is present on neural cell membranes in humans (Johnson, Bailey, & Mobraaten, 1981). There are, not surprisingly, alternative (and occasionally credible) explanations for virtually every natural or clinical phenomenon that has been described thus far or will be described below. Still, it is the author's opinion that the theory has an appeal, and perhaps also a certain usefulness.

Hypotheses Engendered by the Theory

The Immunoreactive Theory and the structure of sex differences on which it is based are particularly interesting in light of the hypotheses they engender. It is likely that many of the hypotheses presented below can be tested in existing data sets.

Parity Effects

The Immunoreactive Theory is derived, in part, from the demonstration of negative parity effects in at least some of the developmental disorders. But it does not require nor does it predict that parity effects will be found for all psychiatric, neurologic, and developmental disorders. The birth order/parity literature with respect to specific psychiatric and neurologic disorders (e.g., schizophrenia, epilepsy, alcoholism) is extensive but inconsistent, and there are serious methodological difficulties in executing a definitive parity study in clinical populations.

Because birth order effects are relatively slight, large numbers of subjects are required to detect them (Birtchnell, 1971). Birth order studies rarely compare their findings to a general population control group, and the statistical analysis that is most often used, the Greenwood-Yule method, is not without its critics (McKeown & Record, 1956). Birth order effects are sensitive to changes in the birth rate, numbers of marriages, and family size in the general population, and a decrease in family size, for example, may lead to an overrepresentation of early birth ranks in small sibships and an increase in later birth ranks in large sibships (Price & Hare, 1969). To consider sibling position irrespective of the size or composition of the sibship in which it occurs is probably unjustifiable (Birtchnell, 1971). Additional sources of bias that can compromise the findings of a birth order study include the analysis of incomplete sibships, differential survival by birth rank, differential migration to sources of ascertainment of patients (Hare & Price, 1969), and the fact that birth order does not necessarily agree with pregnancy order (Metrakos & Metrakos, 1963). Parity studies of psychiatric disorders may be compromised by the fact that death, divorce, separation, or other causes of early parental loss cannot prevent the conception of the last child in a family. Accordingly, the likelihood of parental deprivation having occurred during early childhood will always be greater for later born than for earlier born persons (Delint, 1966).

The Primiparity Effect

The deleterious effects of primiparity may obscure a birth order effect. Primiparas are more prone to obstetrical complications, such as dystocia and toxemia. Subfertile women will be overrepresented among primiparas. A woman whose first child is defective has a number of strong reasons to limit the size of her family. Congenital rubella and infantile autism are examples of disorders in which relative risk is greatest for first borns (Deykin & MacMahon, 1980; Schoenbaum, Biano, & Mack, 1975); thereafter, however, a parity effect appears to emerge. A U-shaped distribution of pathologic events with parity has also been described in association with fetal loss after 20 weeks of gestation, stillbirths, and neonatal death (Ernst & Angst, 1983).

The relative risk of rubella and autism may be plotted against birth order. First borns are at greatest risk, but for ensuing birth orders there is a clear parity effect. One suggested way to measure the relationship between parity and risk for these disorders is orthogonal polynominal analysis of variance. When this method is applied to the data contained in cited references (Deykin & MacMahon, 1980; Schoenbaum et al., 1975), it is found that the quadratic relation (i.e., risk declines from birth order 1 to 2, increases thereafter) captures substantially more of the variance in the sample than the linear relation (Rubella: r^2 (linear) $= 0.04$, $F(1,106) = 143.5$; r^2 (quadratic) $= 0.93$, $F(1,106) = 1423.3$; analysis of difference between slopes by Fischer's r to z transform, $z = 13.04$ (150). Autism: r^2 (linear) $= 0.05$, $F(1,455) = 45.86$; r^2 (quadratic) $= 0.46$, $F(1,455) = 417.3$; difference, $z = 4.07$ (151)). The proper analysis of a birth defect has to take this primiparity effect into consideration.

Sex Differences in Parity Effects

Parity effects are more interesting to examine with an eye to specific hypotheses (Ernst & Angst, 1983). If, for example, the question has to do with relative male vulnerability to a negative birth order effect, study of parity effects is enlightening. For example, the author's re-analysis of data from the Second National Health Survey, 1963–65, shows that males are more vulnerable to parity effects than females. The National Health Survey was an epidemiologically sophisticated population survey of 7119 American children aged 6–9 (Roberts & Engel, 1974). One part of the survey was an IQ estimate derived from Vocabulary and Block Design subtests of the Wechsler Intelligence Scale for Children. In this survey, clear parity effects on IQ were found; however, the parity effect was felt more sharply by boys than girls. The slope of the regression line of IQ on birth orders is -2.34 for boys and -1.57 for girls (Orthogonal polynomial regression analysis, sex times birth order (linear), $F(1,7117) = 239.13$, $p = .005$. (After the author had done this analysis, Steelman and Mercy (1983) published the same data set using multiple regression analysis and demonstrated the same effect.

The author's re-analysis of IQ data published in two additional studies confirms the relative susceptibility of male offspring to negative birth order effects. In 1965, Reed and Reed published *Mental Retardation: A Family Study,* an extraordinary and unique collection of pedigree analysis on 289 residents of an institution for mentally retarded persons in Minnesota. Actual IQ scores were available for 258 probands, 118 boys and 140 girls. These were regressed against birth order. The correlation between IQ and birth order for boys was negative ($R = -0.45$, $p = .001$, slope $= -1.5$), while for girls the correlation was actually positive ($R = 0.48$, $p = .001$, slope $= 1.4$) (difference between slopes, $F(1,256) = 37.075$, $p = .0005$).

The data are even more striking in a more homogeneous group of mentally retarded children who had all been born prematurely. These data were re-analyzed from Moore's 1965 study of 137 mentally retarded residents of the Arizona Children's Colony. The correlation between birth order and degree of retardation was again negative for boys ($N = 63$, $r = -0.85$, $p < .001$, slope $= -0.74$) and positive for girls ($N = 71$, $r = 0.93$, $p < .001$, slope $+00.30$) ($F(1,126) = 11.22$, $p < .001$).

It is clear that there is more to parity effects than a simple birth order analysis yields. The sex of the proband is a relevant variable, but it is not usually considered in birth order studies of cognitive development or of neuropsychiatric disorders.

If parity effects are more sharply felt by the male fetus, one should expect to see the birth of developmentally handicapped boys earlier in the sibship. The data of Reed and Reed (1965) and of Moore (1965) provide at least some support for this prediction. The mean birth rank for 137 boys in Reed and Reed was 3.3 (±2.4) and for 152 girls, 3.7 (±2.5). In Moore, the mean birth rank for boys ($N = 63$) was 3.1 (±3.0) and for girls ($N = 71$), 3.3 (±2.5). Although neither result was significant at the 0.05 level, both were in the predicted direction.

Another way to look at parity effects is to examine the sex ratio/parity interaction in special populations. The sex ratio decreases with parity in the general population, as mentioned above, but the decrement is very small (slope $= -0.001$ (Novitski & Sandler, 1956)). The IMRT predicts that the sex ratio/parity regression line will be steeper in developmentally impaired populations because of increased occurrence of maternal immunoreactivity. A comparison of sex ratio/parity lines is given in three populations: the general population from the 1946–52 U.S. Vital Statistics (Novitski & Sandler, 1956); a sample of 496 patients with congenital cleft lip/palate (Woolf, 1971); and 880 siblings and probands from Reed and Reed's study (1965). The regression lines are substantially steeper, by a factor of 30, in the two disordered samples.

Yet another way to analyze parity effects in light of the IMRT is to test the hypothesis that with increasing birth order offspring should increasingly come to resemble their mothers. Having been sensitized by several previous pregnancies, mothers ought to "prefer" antigenically similar zygotes. This hypothesis is guided, of course, by the fact that the sex ratio decreases with parity; i.e., relatively more girls are born later in the sibship. Judging from the very small sex ratio effect, however, it is likely that only a very large data bank will yield a proper answer to this question.

An atheoretical approach to parity effects in psychiatric illness or neurodevelopmental disorders, executed in relatively small and possibly biased samples, is not likely to yield useful information. Within the context of a specific hypothesis, however, such as relative male/female vulnerability or the IMRT, the study of birth order effects can be both interesting and enlightening.

Parity Effects and IQ

The phenomenon of parity effects was first described in 1874 by Francis Galton, who noted a disproportionate number of first-born children among fellows of the Royal Society. Galton was the first modern scientist to suggest that primogeniture conferred a unique and selective advantage on intellectual development. The modern variant is found in studies of parity or birth order effects on intelligence (Belmont & Marolla, 1973). It is reasonably well established that IQ scores of first-borns are higher and that IQ decreases with birth order (Belmont & Marolla, 1973). The effect holds even when maternal age is controlled. This finding has usually been explained in psychosocial terms: parents spend more time with first-born children, they play with them more, they talk to them more, they expect more of them, and so on (Altus, 1966; Galton, 1874; Zajonc, 1976). The family environment of later borns is necessarily shared and diminished. This is an intuitive explanation and one that is given to empirical examination; however, attempts to confirm this hypothesis have not been notably successful (Ernst & Angst, 1983; Grotevant, Scarr, & Weinberg, 1977). For example, socioeconomic advantage and early stimulation mitigates but does not abolish parity effects on IQ (Zajonc,

1983). The family versus environment argument (or *confluence* model) (Zajonc, 1976) predicts that closer spacing of siblings will compound the parity effect; in fact, spacing effects on intellectual development have not been found to exist in developed countries, where close spacing does not lead to maternal undernutrition (Belmont, Stein, & Zybert, 1978; Grotevant et al., 1977).

Negative parity effects are found not only for IQ and academic achievement, which may be amenable to psychosocial explanation, but also for specific learning disabilities (Badian, 1984; Schrag, 1973), mental retardation (Belmont et al., 1976), perinatal mortality (Niswander & Gordon, 1972), and height (Belmont, Stein, & Susser, 1975), which clearly are not. Parity effects have even been observed in newborns (Waldrop & Bell, 1966). The IMRT represents an alternative, biological explanation for negative parity effects in general and it is particularly germane to parity effects on intellectual development.

The Antecedent Brother Effect

The IMRT predicts that parity effects on later born boys will be greater if antecedent siblings are boys. In such cases, mothers may be sensitized to H-Y antigen or to other sex-linked antigens. This sensitization can compromise the development of subsequent male fetuses. The idea is borrowed from studies of the sex ratio and of placentation relative to antecedent brothers (*vide supra*). The antecedent brother hypothesis can be tested by comparing relative parity effects on any neurodevelopmental measure in males with antecedent brothers against males with antecedent sisters. Crossed comparisons can also be made with females who have antecedent brothers or sisters.

In a study of college entrance examination scores in 1,013 students (Rosenberg & Sutton-Smith, 1969), second-born females scored the same as or higher than first-born females. Boys with older sisters scored higher than boys with older brothers. The data in this paper, however, were not sufficient to allow a statistical re-analysis.

Additional statistical support for the antecedent brother hypothesis was available, however, in Breland's study of 794,589 11th grade students who took the National Merit Scholarship Qualifying Test in 1965 (Breland, 1974). In the author's re-analysis of these data, four family configurations were compared: males with antecedent brothers, males with antecedent sisters, females with antecedent brothers, and females with antecedent sisters. Negative parity effects were seen for all four groups, but the sharpest negative parity effect was observed in boys with antecedent brothers (Gualtieri & Hicks, 1985b).

These two data sets contain selected populations, college-bound high school students and college freshmen, who are not representative of the population as a whole. The fact that these students were at least 16 years old introduces the possibility that psychosocial factors may have played a role in the development of younger children from same-sexed sibships, although the authors are not aware of a convincing psychosocial explanation for such an effect.

The antecedent brother hypothesis could conceivably be tested in large populations relative to any intellectual, developmental, or neuropathic measure. It could also be tested in deviant populations: in mentally retarded children, for example, the hypothesis predicts that increased severity of retardation will occur in males who have antecedent brothers as compared with males who have antecedent sisters. The antecedent brother effect may also play a role in some other hypotheses derived from the IMRT, as described below.

Subfertility

If maternal immunoreactivity is related to development disorders, one may expect to see relative infertility in the families of developmentally disabled children. Relative infertility can be measured indirectly by family size or directly by the length of time required for unprotected mothers to conceive. In fact, relative infertililty has been found in mothers of children with mental retardation (Wallace, 1974), Down syndrome (Tips, Smith, & Meyer, 1964), cerebral palsy (Tips et al., 1964), epilepsy (Drillien, 1968), congenital anomalies (Drillien, 1968), learning problems (Nichols & Chen, 1981) and low birth weight (Wilson, Parmelee, & Huggins, 1963). This effect is even more pronounced when the disordered child is male (Wallace, 1974). There is as a rule a longer period of relative infertility after the birth of male children in general (Wyshak, 1969). The sex ratio of children born to relatively infertile mothers favors the birth of girls (James, 1985).

The IMRT predicts not only that relative infertility should characterize mothers of developmentally disabled children, but also that the phenomenon should be more apparent when the disabled child is a boy. This prediction was supported by at least one study of children with febrile seizures (Bernard, 1977). A re-analysis of Reed and Reed (1965) revealed that mentally retarded males tend to come from smaller families (males, mean family size 6.1; females 7.0; $t = 2.12$, $p = 0.02$, one-tailed test). Maternal immunoreactivity may contribute to the birth of a fetus who is developmentally retarded and may also lower fertility thereafter.

Studies of maternal subfertility and reproductive inefficiency support the IMRT, but further studies with much larger samples should be done.

Additional Hypotheses

The IMRT predicts that antigenic dissimilarity would increase the likelihood of maternal immune attack upon the fetus. When a developmentally handicapped child is born in a large sibship, it is hypothesized that he will be more likely to differ from his mother in measurable antigenic characteristics such as HLA or ABO. It is also predicted that there will be a tendency for later born sibs to resemble their mothers more closely in terms of the same antigenic characteristics. It is also proposed that antigenically dissimilar matings will be prone to produce female offspring. These hypotheses are based on the premise that H-Y and other antigen systems exercise an additive effect. They could conceivably be tested in the data banks that are maintained by tissue transplant services where typing records are maintained on families.

The IMRT is premised on the idea of an immunoreactive subgroup of mothers. It predicts that such immunoreactive mothers will exhibit an increased incidence of infertility and maternal insufficiency. It is possible that such women may be identified by the presence of allergic or autoimmune disorders. The occurrence of maternal insufficiency in women with autoimmune disease has been reviewed above. It is proposed that allergic and autoimmune disorders will occur more commonly in the mothers of developmentally handicapped children, in their families, and in the children themselves.

In fact, a frequent complaint of the parents of developmentally disabled children is their proneness to allergies. Although this has never received much attention from clinicians or researchers, recent studies have shown patterns of abnormal immmunoresponsivity in children with infantile autism and Down syndrome (Fialkow, 1966; Stubbs, 1976; Stubbs & Crawford, 1977; Weizman, Weizman, Szekely, Wijsenbeek, & Levni, 1982). The IMRT predicts that mothers of such children would include a substantial number of immunoreactive individuals; this factor could contribute to their children's disabilities. In support, abnormal levels of immunoreactivity have been reported in the families of children with Down syndrome (Fialkow, 1966). Geschwind's recent report of an increased occurrence of autoimmune disorders in left-handers and their families is also consistent with this line of thinking, although in that study no distinction was made between familial and pathological sinistrals (Geschwind & Behan, 1982). The latter would be expected to exhibit the trait more strongly. It is not unreasonable to suggest that a genetic disposition to autoimmune or allergic disorders might be associated with heightened maternal immunoreactivity and left-handedness may simply be one more clinical consequence thereof.

Clinicians who work with developmentally handicapped children will occasionally come upon families who exhibit this pattern: the first child is normal; the second, learning disabled; and the third, retarded or autistic. Such families represent an ideal *immunoreactive subgroup* for further investigation. Mothers whose children follow such a pattern would be expected to be especially immunoreactive, might also be expected to have strong family histories of immunoreactivity, and might also be expected to have strong family histories of immunoreactive disorders. Hypotheses concerning specific kinds of immune activity connected with maternal-fetal attack would best be tested in such a subgroup.

Finally, a far-fetched idea, but one that is intriguing and irresistable to the author, at least, in light of the foregoing. There seems to be a unique and truly remarkable association between fetal sex and schizophrenia occurring in pregnancy. In 1967, Shearer, Davidson, and Finch reported that only female children had been born to women who conceived within one month before or after an acute schizophrenic episode. This finding was later confirmed by Taylor (1969), who also reported four stillbirths (all males), two perinatal deaths (both males), and six severe birth defects (five of the six males) in mothers who became psychotic during the second or third month of pregnancy. It was suggested that there is a *factor* in acutely psychotic mothers that is especially toxic to the male embryo (Shearer et al., 1967). This element could be hormonal, but, in light of some recent autoimmune theories of schizophrenia, it could also be immunologic. Perhaps the element is the initiation of an acute hyperimmune state provoked by the fetus leading to maternal attack not only against fetal tissue, but also against her own brain tissue. Of course there is no direct evidence to support this idea. But it is not outlandish to suggest that hypotheses germane to the IMRT might be profitably tested in schizophrenics, or at least in schizophrenics with early onset or evidence of neuropathic damage.

SUMMARY

The IMRT draws from a diverse array of sources to present a possible etiology for many cases of neurodevelopmental impairment. It is concerned with the problems of selective male affliction, maternal insufficiency, the structure of sex differences, and negative parity effects on intellectual development. The strongest appeal of the theory lies neither in its internal consistency nor in its success in bringing together obscure and seemingly unrelated findings, but rather in its ability to engender testable hypotheses. Many of these are affirmed in the literature or by preliminary investigations derived from existing data.

The theory suggests two interesting routes for further investigation, the antecedent brother effect and the study of immunoreactive subgroups.

It is strongly suggested that studies of parity effects, pre- and perinatal complications, maternal insufficiency, and family genetic background relative to intellectual development take into consideration the sex of the proband and of antecedent siblings and the family proclivity to autoimmune and to allergic disorders.

If the theory were supported by research along the lines suggested above, hypotheses concerning specific immunologic mechanisms might be developed. Such research might yield strategies for the prevention of some of the neurodevelopmental disorders of childhood.

REFERENCES

Aarkrog, T. (1968). Organic factors in infantile psychoses: Retrospective study of 46 cases subjected to pneumoencephalography. *Danish Medical Bulletin, 15,* 283–288.

Abramowicz, H.K., & Richardson, S.A. (1975). Epideminology of severe mental retardation in children. *American Journal on Mental Deficiency, 80,* 18–39.

Abramsky, O., Lisalc, R.P., Silberger, D.H., & Pleasure, D.E. (1977). Antibodies to oligodendroglia in patients with multiple schlerosis. *New England Journal of Medicine, 297,* 1207–1211.

Abramsky, O., & Litvin, Y. (1978). Autoimmune response to dopamine-receptor as a possible mechanism in the pathogenesis of Parkinson's disease and schizophrenia. *Perspectives in Biology and Medicine, 22,* 104–114.

Adinolfi, M. (1976). Neurologic handicap and permeability of the blood-CSF barrier during fetal life to maternal antibodies and hormones. *Developmental Medicine and Child Neurology, 18,* 243–246.

Adinolfi, M., Beck, S.E., Haddad, S.A., & Seller, M.J. (1976). Permeability of the blood-CSF barrier to plasma proteins during foetal and perinatal life. *Nature, 259,* 140–141.

Ahern, F.M., & Johnson, R.C. (1973). Inherited uterine inadequacy: An alternative explanation for a portion of cases of defect. *Behavior Genetics, 3,* 1–12.

Allon, R. (1971). Sex, race, socioeconomic status, social mobility, and process-reactive ratings of schizophrenics. *Journal of Nervous and Mental Disorders, 153,* 343–350.

Altus, W.D. (1966). Birth order and its sequellae. *Science, 151,* 441–459.

August, G.J., Stewart, M.A., & Tsai, L. (1981). The incidence of cognitive disabilities in the siblings of autistic children. *British Journal of Psychiatry, 138,* 416–422.

Badian, N. (1984). Reading disability in an epidemiologic context: Incidence and environmental correlates. *Journal of Learning Disabilities, 17,* 129–136.

Bakketeig, L.S. (1977). The risk of repeated preterm or low birth weight delivery. In D. M. Reed & F.J. Stanley (Eds.), *The Epidemiology of Prematurity* (pp. 231–241). Baltimore: Urban and Schwarzenberg.

Bardawil, W.A., Mitchell, G.W., McKeogh, R.P., & Marchant, D.J. (1962). Behaviour of skin homografts in human pregnancy. I. Habitual abortion. *American Journal of Obstetrics and Gynecology, 84,* 1283–1295.

Barnes, R.D., & Tuffrey, M. (1971). Maternal cells in the newborn. *Advances in Biosciences, 6,* 457–473.

Beck, J.S., & Rowell, N.R. (1963). Transplacental passage of antinuclear antibody. *Lancet, I,* 134–135.

Beer, A.E., & Billingham, R.E. (1973). Maternally acquired runt disease. *Science, 179,* 240–245.

Belmont, L., & Marolla, F.A. (1973). Birth order, family size and intelligence. *Science, 182,* 1096–1101.

Belmont, L., Stein, Z.A., & Susser, M.W. (1975). Comparisons of associations of birth order with intelligence test score and height. *Nature, 255,* 54–55.

Belmont, L., Stein, Z.A., & Wittes, J.A. (1976). Birth order, family size and school failure. *Developmental Medicine and Child Neurology, 18,* 421–430.

Belmont, L., Stein, Z., & Zybert, P. (1978). Child spacing and birth order: Effects of intellectual ability in two-child families. *Science, 202,* 995–996.

Bernard, O. (1977). Possible protecting role of maternal immunoglobulins on embryonic development in mammals. *Immunogenetics, 5,* 1–15.

Berryman, P.L., & Silvers, W.K. (1979). Studies on the H-X locus of mice. *Immunogenetics, 9,* 363–367.

Billingham, R.E. (1964). Transplantation immunity and the maternal-fetal relationship. *New England Journal of Medicine, 270,* 667–672; 720–725.

Birtchnell, J. (1971). Mental illness in sibships of two and three. *British Journal of Psychiatry, 119,* 481–487.

Blessing, W.W., Costa, M., Gefen, L.B., & Rush, R.A. (1977). Immune lesions of noradrenergic neurons in rat central nervous system produced by antibodies to dopamine-B-hydroxylase. *Nature, 167,* 368–369.

Bonner, J.J., Terasaki, P.L., Thompson, R., Holve, L.M., Wilson, L., Ebbin, A.J., & Slavkin, H.C. (1978). HLA phenotype frequencies in individuals with cleft lip and/or cleft palate. *Tissue Antigens, 12,* 228–232.

Borland, R., Loke, Y.W., & Oldersnaw, P.J. (1970). Sex differences in trophoblast behavior on transplantation. *Nature, 228,* 572.

Breland, H. (1974). Birth order, family configuration and verbal achievement. *Child Development, 45,* 1011–1019.

Brent, L. (1971). The effect of immune reactions on fetal development. *Advances in Biosciences, 6,* 421–455.

Bresnihan, B., Grigor, R.R., Oliver, M., Leiskomia, R.M., & Hughes, G.R.V. (1977). Immunological mechanism for spontaneous abortion in systemic lupus erythematosis. *Lancet, V,* 1205–1207.

Burbaeva, G.S. (1972). Antigen characteristics of the human brain. *Soviet Neurology and Psychiatry, 5,* 110–118.

Burgio, G.R., Fraccaro, M., Ticpolo, L., & Wolf, U. (1981). *Trisomy 21.* Berlin: Springer-Verlag.

Burke, J., & Johansen, K. (1974). The formation of HL-A antibodies in pregnancy. The antigenicity of aborted and term fetuses. *Journal of Obstetrics and Gynecology in the British Commonwealth, 81,* 222–228.

Butler, N.R., & Bonham, D.G. (1963). *Perinatal Mortality.* Edinburgh: Churchill Livingstone.

Cadoret, R.J., & Cain, C. (1980). Sex differences in prediction of antisocial behavior in adoptees. *Archives of General Psychiatry, 37,* 1171–1175.

Carter, C.O. (1965). The inheritance of common congential malformation. *Progress in Medical Genetics, 4,* 59–84.

Chesley, L.C., Annito, J.E., & Cosgrove, R.A. (1968). The familial factor in toxemia of pregnancy. *Obstetrics and Gynecology, 32,* 303–311.

Childs, B. (1965). Genetic origin of some sex differences among human beings. *Pediatrics, 35,* 798–812.

Ciocco, A. (1940). Sex differences in morbidity and mortality. *Quarterly Review of Biology, 15,* 59–92.

Clarke, B., & Kirby, D.R.S. (1966). Maintenance of histocompatability polymorphisms. *Nature, 211,* 999–1000.

Cloninger, C.R., Christiansen, K.O., Reich, T., & Gottesman, I.I. (1978). Implications of sex differences in the prevalences of antisocial personality, alcoholism, and criminality for familial transmission. *Archives of General Psychiatry, 35,* 941–951.

Cohen, B.H., & Mellitts, E.D. (1971). Blood group incompatibility and immunoglobulin levels. *Johns Hopkins Medical Journal, 128,* 318–331.

Corbett, J.A., Harris, R., & Robinson, R.G. (1975). *Epilepsy in mental retardation and developmental disorders* (Vol. 7, pp. 79–111). New York: Brunner-Mazel.

Costeff, H., Cohen, B.E., & Weller, L.E. (1983). Biological factors in mild mental retardation. *Developmental Medicine and Child Neurology, 25,* 580–587.

Costeff, H., Cohen, B.E., Weller, L., & Kleckner, H. (1981). Pathogenic factors in idiopathic mental retardation. *Developmental Medicine and Child Neurology, 23,* 484–493.

Dalakas, M.C., & Engel, W.K. (1981). Chronic relapsing (dysimmune) polyneuropathy: Pathogenesis and treatment. *Annals of Neurology, 9 (Suppl.),* 134–135.

Decker, S.N., & DeFries, J.C. (1980). Cognitive abilities in families of reading-disabled children. *Journal of Learning Disabilities, 13,* 517–522.

Dekaban, A.S., & Sadowsky, D. (1978). Changes in brain weights during the span of human life. *Annals of Neurology, 4,* 345–356.

Delint, J.E.E. (1966). The position of early parental loss in the etiology of alcoholism. *Alcoholism Zagreb, 2,* 56–64.

Deykin, E.Y., & MacMahon, B. (1980). Pregnancy, delivery and neonatal complications among autistic children. *American Journal of Diseases of Children, 134,* 860–864.

Doughty, R.W., & Gelsthorpe, K. (1974). An initial investigation of lymphocyte antibody activity through pregnancy and in eluates prepared from placental material. *Tissue Antigens, 4,* 291–298.

Doughty, R.W., & Gelsthorpe, K. (1976). Some parameters of lymphocyte antibody activity through pregnancy and further eluates of placental material. *Tissue Antigens, 8,* 43–48.

Drillien, C.M. (1968). Studies in mental handicap II: Some obstetric factors of possible aetiological significance. *Archives of Disease in Childhood, 43,* 283–294.

Eichwald, E.J., & Silmser, C.R. (1955). *Transplantation Bulletin, 2,* 148–149.

Ernst, C., & Angst, J. (1983). *Birth order: Its influence on personality.* Berlin: Springer-Verlag.

Fabia, J., & Drolette, M. (1970). Life tables up to age 10 for mongols with and without congential heart disease. *Journal of Mental Deficiency Research, 14,* 235.

Farber, C., Cambiaso, C.L., & Masson, P.L. (1981). Immune complexes in cord serum. *Clinical and Experimental Immunology , 44,* 426–432.

Fialkow, P.J. (1966). Autoimmunity and chromosomal aberrations. *American Journal of Human Genetics, 18,* 93–108.

Flor-Henry, P. (1969). Psychosis and temporal lobe epilepsy: A controlled investigation. *Epilepsia, 10,* 363.

Flor-Henry, P. (1974). Psychosis, neurosis and epilepsy: Developmental and gender related effects. *British Journal of Psychiatry, 124,* 144–150.

Forssman, H., & Akesson, J.O. (1970). Mortality of the mentally deficient: A study of 12,903 institutionalized subjects. *Journal of Mental Deficiency Research, 4,* 276.

Foster, J.W., & Archer, S.J. (1979). Birth order and intelligence: An immunological interpretation. *Perceptual and Motor Skills, 48,* 79–93.

Funderburk, S.J., Carter, J., Tanguay, P., Freeman, B.J., & Westlake, J.R. (1983). Parental reproductive problems and gestational hormone exposure in autistic and schizophrenic children. *Journal of Autism and Developmental Disabilities, 13,* 325–332.

Galton, F. (1874). *English men of science: Their nature and nurture.* London: Macmillan.

Gardner, C.G. (1967). Role of maternal psychopathology in male and female schizophrenics. *Journal of Consulting Psychology, 31,* 411–413.

Garside, R.F., & Kay, D.W.K. (1964). The genetics of stuttering. In G. Andrews & M.M. Harris (Eds.). *The syndrome of stuttering.* London: Heinemann.

Geschwind, N., & Behan, P. (1982). Left-handedness: Association with immune disease, migraine and developmental learning disorder. *Proceedings of the National Academy of Science of the USA, 79,* 5097–5100.

Gillberg, C., & Gillberg, I.C. (1983). Infantile autism: A total population study of reduced optimality in the pre-, peri-, and neonatal period. *Journal of Autism and Developmental Disabilities, 13,* 153–166.

Gillberg, C., & Rasmussen, P. (1982). Perceptual, motor and attentional deficits in seven-year-old children: Background factors. *Developmental Medicine and Child Neurology, 24,* 752–770.

Gleicher, N., & Siegel, I. (1980). The immunologic concept of EPH-Gestosis. *Mt. Sinai Journal of Medicine, 47,* 442–453.

Glucksmann, A. (1978). *Sex determination and sexual dimorphism in mammals.* London: Wykeham.

Goodfellow, P.N., & Andrews, P.W. (1982). Sexual differentiation and H-Y antigen. *Nature, 295,* 11–13.
Goulmy, E., Termijtelen, A., Bradley, B.A., & Van Rood, J.J. (1977). Y-antigen killing by T cells of women is restricted by HL-A. *Nature, 266,* 544–545.
Graham, P., & Rutter, M. (1968). Organic brain dysfunction and child psychiatric disorder. *British Medical Journal, 3,* 695–700.
Grotevant, H.D., Scarr, S., & Weinberg, R.A. (1977). Intellectual development in family constellations with natural and adopted children: A test of the Zajonc & Markus model. *Child Development, 48,* 1699–1703.
Grotevant, H.D., Scarr, S., & Weinberg, R.A. (1983). Intellectual development in family conperiod. *Journal of Autism and Developmental Disabilities, 13,* 153–166.
Gualtieri, C.T. (1983). Unpublished data.
Gualtieri, C.T., & Hicks, R.E. (1985a). ABO incompatibility and parity effects on perinatal mortality. *Social Biology, 32*(1–2), 129–131.
Gualtieri, C.T., & Hicks, R.E. (1985b). Parity effects on intellectual development are influenced by sex of antecedent siblings. Manuscript submitted.
Gualtieri, C.T., & Hicks, R.E. (1985c). An immunoreactive theory of selective male affliction. *Behavioral and Brain Sciences, 8*(3), 427–477.
Gualtieri, C.T., Hicks, R.E., & Mayo, R.P. (1984). Influence of sex of antecedent siblings on human sex ratio. *Life Sciences, 34,* 1791–1794.
Hagberg, B., Hagberg, G., Lewerth, A., & Linberg, V. (1981). Mild mental retardation in Swedish school children. II: Etiologic and pathogenetic aspects. *Acta Paediatrica Scandinavica, 70,* 445–452.
Halbrecht, I., & Komlos, L. (1976). E-rosette-forming lymphocytes in mother and new-born. *Lancet, I,* 544.
Hare, E.H., & Price, J.S. (1969). Birth order and family size: Bias caused by changes in birth rate. *British Journal of Psychiatry, 115,* 647–656.
Harris, R.E., & London, R.E. (1976). The association of maternal lymphocytotoxic antibodies with obstetric complications. *Obstetrics and Gynecology, 48,* 302–304.
Hauser, S.L., Dawson, D.M., Lehrich, J.R., Beal, M.F., Kevy, S.V., Propper, R.D., Mills, J.A., & Weiner, H.L. (1983). Intensive immunosuppression in progressive multiple schlerosis. *New England Journal of Medicine, 308,* 173–180.
Hicks, R.E., & Gualtieri, C.T. (1985). The structure of sex differences in developmental handicap. Manuscript submitted.
Hicks, R.E., & Kinsbourne, M. (1981). Fathers and sons, mothers and children: A note on the sex effect on left-handedness. *Journal of Genetic Psychology, 139,* 305–306.
Hutt, C. (1972). Neuroendocrinological, behavioral and intellectual aspects of sexual differentiation in human development. In C. Ounsted & D.C. Taylor (Eds.), *Gender differences: Their ontogeny and significance* (pp. 73–122). Edinburgh: Churchill Livingstone.
Ingram, T.T.S. (1959). Specific developmental disorders of speech in childhood. *Brain, 82,* 450–467.
Ingram, T.T.S. (1964). *Pediatric aspects of cerebral palsy.* London: Churchill Livingstone.
James, D.A. (1965). Effects of antigenic dissimilarity between mother and foetus of placental size in mice. *Nature, 205,* 613–614.
James, W.M. (1985). The sex ratio of infants born after hormonal induction of ovulation. *British Journal of Obstetrics and Gynecology, 92,* 299–301.
Joffe, J.M. (1969). *Prenatal determinants of behavior.* Oxford: Pergamon Press.
Johansen, K., & Burke, J. (1974). Possible relationships between maternal HL-A antibody formation and fetal sex. *Journal of Obstetrics and Gynecology in the British Commonwealth, 81,* 781–785.
Johansen, K., Festenstein, H., & Burke, J. (1974). Possible relationships between maternal HL-A antibody formation and fetal sex. Evidence for a sex-linked histocompatibility system in man. *Journal of Obstetrics and Gynecology in the British Commonwealth, 81,* 781–785.
Johnson, E.M., Gorin, P.D., Brandeis, L.D., & Pearson, J. (1980). Dorsal root ganglion neurons are destroyed by exposure in utero to maternal antibody to nerve growth factor. *Science, 210,* 916–918.

Johnson, L.L., Bailey, D.W., & Mobraaten, L.E. (1981). Genetics of histocompatibility in mice. IV. Detection of certain minor (non-Hz) H antigens in selected organs by the popliteal node test. *Immunogenetics, 14*, 63–71.
Jones, W.R. (1968). Immunological factors in human placentation. *Nature, 218*, 480.
Keller, C.A. (1981). Epidemiological characteristics of preterm births. In S.L. Friedman & M. Sigman (Eds.), *Preterm birth and psychological development*. New York: Academic Press.
Kirby, D.R.S., McWhirter, K.G., Teitelbaum, M.S., & Darlington, C.D. (1967). A possible immunologic influence on sex ratio. *Lancet II*, 139–140.
Kitzmiller, J.L. (1978). Autoimmune disorders: Maternal, fetal and neonatal risks. *Clinical Obstetrics and Gynecology, 21*, 385–396.
Kolyaskina, G.I., Boehme, D.I., Buravlev, V.M., & Faktor, M.I. (1977). Certain aspects of the study of the brain of the human embryo. *Soviet Neurology and Psychiatry, 10*, 24–31.
Kramer, M. (1978). Population changes and schizophrenia, 1970–1985. In L. Wynne, R. Cromwell, & S. Mathysse (Eds.), *The Nature of Schizophrenia: New Approaches* (pp. 545–571). New York: Wiley.
Krco, C.J., & Goldberg, E.H. (1976). H-Y (male) antigen: Detection on 8-cell embryos. *Science, 193*, 1134–1135.
Lawler, S.D., Ukaejoofo, E.D., & Reeves, B.R. (1975). Interaction between maternal and neonatal cells in mixed-lymphocyte cultures. *Lancet I*, 1185–1186.
Lehrke, R.G. (1978). Sex linkage: A biological basis for greater male variability in intelligence. In R.T. Osborne, C.E. Noble, & N. Weyl (Eds.), *Human Variation* (Vol. 1, pp. 171–198). New York: Academic Press.
Lewitter, F.I., DeFries, J.C., & Elston, R.C. (1980). Genetic models of reading disability. *Behavior Genetics, 10*, 9–30.
Lilienfield, A.M., & Pasamanick, B. (1956). The association of maternal and fetal factors with the development of mental deficiency. II: Relationship to maternal age, birth order, previous reproductive loss and degree of maternal deficiency. *American Journal of Mental Deficiency, 60*, 557–569.
Loke, Y.W. (1978). *Immunology and immunopathology of the human fetal-maternal interaction.* Amsterdam: Elsevier.
Lord, C., Schopler, E., & Revicki, D. (1982). Sex differences in autism. *Journal of Autism and Developmental Disorders, 12*, 317–330.
Lotter, V. (1970). Factors related to outcome in autistic children. *Journal of Autism and Childhood Schizophrenia, 4*, 263–277.
Maccoby, E.E., Doering, C.H., Jacklin, C.N., & Kraemer, H. (1979). Concentrations of sex hormones in umbilical-cord blood: Their relation to sex and birth order of infants. *Child Development, 50*, 632–642.
McGlone, J. (1980). Sex differences in human brain asymmetry: A critical survey. *Behavioral and Brain Sciences, 3*, 215–263.
McKeown, T., & Record, R.G. (1956). Maternal age and birth order as indices of environmental influence. *American Journal of Human Genetics, 8*, 8–23.
McKinney, D., & Feagans, L. (1983). Unpublished data.
McLaren, A. (1962). Does maternal immunity to male antigen affect the sex ratio of the young? *Nature, 195*, 1323–1324.
McMillen, M.M. (1979). Differential mortality by sex in fetal and neonatal deaths. *Science, 204*, 89–91.
McPherson, C.F.C. (1970). Immunochemical approaches to the study of brain function and psychiatric diseases. *Canadian Psychiatric Association Journal, 15*, 641–645.
Medawar, P.B. (1963). Some immunological and endocrinological problems raised by the evolution of viviparity in vertebrates. In *Symposia of the Society for Experimental Biology*, Symposium No. 9, pp. 320–338. New York: Academic Press.
Mednick, S.A. (1970). Breakdown in individuals at high risk for schizophrenia: Possible predispositional perinatal factors. *Mental Hygiene, 54*, 50–63.
Mednick, S.A., Mura, E., Schulsinger, F., & Mednick, B. (1971). Perinatal conditions and infant development in children with schizophrenic parents. *Social Biology, 18*, 103–113.
Mednick, S.A., Schulsinger, F., Teasdale, T.W., Schulsinger, H., Venables, P.H., & Rock, D.R. (1977). Schizophrenia in high risk children: Sex differences in predisposing factors.

In G. Serban (Ed.), *Cognitive defects in the development of mental illness.* New York: Brunner/Mazel.

Metrakos, J.D., & Metrakos, K. (1963). Is pregnancy order a factor in epilepsy? *Journal of Neurology, Neurosurgery and Psychiatry, 26,* 451–457.

Mizuno, M., Lobotsky, J., Lloyd, C.W., Kobayashi, T., & Murasawa, Y. (1968). Plasma androstenedione and testosterone during pregnancy and in the newborn. *Journal of Clinical Endocrinology and Metabolism, 28,* 1133–1142.

Moore, B.C. (1965). Relationship between prematurity and intelligence in mental retardates. *American Journal of Mental Deficiency, 70,* 448–453.

Nakano, K.K. (1973). Anencephaly: A review. *Developmental Medicine and Child Neurology, 15,* 383.

Nichols, P.L., & Chen T.C. (1981). *Minimal brain dysfunction: A prospective study.* Hillsdale, NJ: Erlbaum.

Niswander, K.R., & Gordon, M. (1972). *The women and their pregnancies.* Philadelphia: Saunders.

Novitski, E. (1977). *Human genetics.* New York: Macmillan.

Novitski, E., & Sandler, L. (1956). The relationship between parental age, birth order and the secondary sex ratio in humans. *Annals of Human Genetics, 21,* 123–31.

Ohama, K., & Kadotani, T. (1971). Lymphocyte reaction in mixed wife-husband leukocyte cultures in relation to infertility. *American Journal of Obstetrics and Gynecology, 109,* 477–479.

Ohno, S. (1979). *Major sex-determining genes.* Berlin: Springer-Verlag.

Ounsted, C., & Ounsted, M. (1970). Effect of Y chromosome on fetal growth rate. *Lancet, II,* 857–858.

Ounsted, C. & Taylor, D.C. (1972). The Y chromosome message: A point of view. In C. Ounsted & D.C. Taylor (Eds.), *Gender differences: Their ontogeny and significance* (pp. 241–262). London: Churchill Livingstone.

Ounsted, M. (1972). Gender and intrauterine growth. In C. Ounsted, & D.C. Taylor (Eds.), *Gender differences: Their ontogeny and significance* (pp. 177–201). London: Churchill Livingstone.

Pennington, B.F., & Smith, S.D. (1983). Genetic influences of learning disabilities and speech and language disorders. *Child Development, 54,* 369–387.

Placek, P. (1977). Maternal and infant health factors associated with low infant birth weight: Findings from the 1972 National Natality Survey. In D.M. Reed & F.J. Stanley (Eds.), *The epidemiology of prematurity* (pp. 197–212). Baltimore: Urban and Schwarzenberg.

Poduslo, S.E., McFarland, H.F., & McKahanon, G.M. (1977). Antiserums to neurons and to oligodendroglia from mammalian brain. *Science, 197,* 270–272.

Price, J.S., & Hare, E.H. (1969). Birth order studies: Some sources of bias. *British Journal of Psychiatry, 115,* 633–646.

Reed, E.W., & Reed, S.C. (1965). *Mental retardation. A family study.* Philadelphia: Saunders.

Reinisch, J.M., Gandelman, R., & Spiegel, F.S. (1979). Prenatal influences on cognitive abilities: Data from experimental animals and human genetic and endocrine studies. In M.A. Wittig & A.C. Petersen (Eds.), *Sex-related differences in cognitive functioning* (pp. 215–240). New York: Academic Press.

Renkonen, K.O., Makela, O., & Lehtovaara, R. (1962). Factors affecting the human sex ratio. *Nature, 194,* 308–309.

Renkonen, K.O., & Timonen, S. (1967). Factors influencing the immunization of Rh-negative mothers. *Journal of Medical Genetics, 4,* 166–168.

Rhodes, P. (1965). Sex of the fetus in antepartum hemmorhage. *Lancet II,* 718–719.

Roberts, J., & Engel, R. (1974). *Family background, early development and intelligence of children 6–11 years.* United States Data from the National Health Survey, DHEW Public #(HRA) 75-1624. Rockville, MD: U.S. Dept. of Health, Education and Welfare, PHS.

Robins, L. (1966). *Deviant children grown up.* Baltimore: Williams & Wilkins.

Robson, E.B. (1955). Birth weight in cousins. *Annals of Human Genetics, 19,* 262–268.

Rosenberg, B.G., & Sutton-Smith, B. (1969). Sibling age spacing effects upon cognition. *Developmental Psychology, 1,* 661–668.

Rosenthal, D. (1962). Familial concordance by sex with respect to schizophrenia. *Psychological Bulletin, 59,* 401–421.
Roszkowski, W., Plaut, M., & Lichtenstein, L.M. (1977). Selective display of histamine receptors on lymphocytes. *Science, 195,* 383–385.
Rubenstein, A. (1982). An immunologic hypothesis concerning some congenital diseases and malformations. *Medical Hypotheses, 9,* 417–419.
Rutter, M. (1970). Sex differences in children's response to family stress. In E.J. Anthony & C. Koupernik (Eds.), *International Yearbook of Child Psychiatry* (pp. 165–196). New York: Wiley.
Sabin, A.B., Krumbiegel, E.R., & Wigand, R. (1958). Echo type 9 virus disease. *American Journal of Diseases of Children, 96,* 197–219.
Samuels, L. (1979). Reply to Lewine. *Schizophrenia Bulletin 5,* 5–10.
Schlesinger, E.R., Alaway, N.C., & Peltin, S. (1959). Survivorship in cerebral palsy. *American Journal of Public Health, 49,* 343.
Schoenbaum, S., Biano, S., & Mack, T. (1975). Epidemiology of congenital rubella syndrome: The role of maternal parity. *Journal of the American Medical Association, 233,* 151–155.
Schrag, H.L. (1973). Program planning for the developmentally disabled: Using survey results. *Mental Retardation, 11,* 8–10.
Scott, J.S. (1976). Immunological aspects of trophoblast neoplasia. In J.S. Scott & W.R. Jones (Eds.), *Immunology of Human Reproduction* (pp. 329–348). New York: Grune & Stratton.
Scott, J.R., & Beer, A.E. (1973). Immunologic factors in first pregnancy Rh immunisation. *Lancet, I,* 717–718.
Scott, J.S., Maddison, P.J., Taylor, P.V., Esschor, E., Scott, D., & Skinner, R.P. (1983). Connective tissue disease, antibodies to ribo-nucleoprotein and congenital heart block. *New England Journal of Medicine, 309,* 209–212.
Sedlis, A., Berendes, H., Kim, H.S., Stone, D.F., Weiss, W., Deutschberger, J., & Jackson, E. The placental weight-birthweight relationship. *Developmental Medicine and Child Neurology, 9,* 160–171.
Shaffer, D., & Fisher, P. (1981). Suicide in children and adolescents. *Journal of the American Academy of Child Psychiatry, 20,* 545–565.
Shearer, M.L., Davidson, R.T., & Finch, S.M. (1967). The sex ratio of offspring born to state hospitalized schizophrenic women. *Journal of Psychiatric Research, 5,* 349–350.
Siiteri, P.K., Febres, F., Clemens, L.E., Chang, R.J., Gondos, B., & Stites, D. (1977). Progesterone and the maintenance of pregnancy: Is progesterone nature's immunosupressant? *Annals of the New York Academy of Science, 286,* 384–397.
Simmons, R.L. (1971). Viviparity, histocompatibility and fetal survival. *Advances in Biosciences, 6,* 405–419.
Singer, J.E., Westphal, M., & Niswander, K.R. (1968). Sex differences in the incidence of neonatal abnormalities and abnormal performance in early childhood. *Child Development, 39,* 103–112.
Slater, E., Beard, A.W., & Glithero, E. (1963). The schizophrenia-like psychoses of epilepsy. *British Journal of Psychiatry, 109,* 95.
Sobel, D.E. (1961). Children of schizophrenic patients: Preliminary observations on early development. *American Journal of Psychiatry, 118,* 512–517.
Sotelo, J., Gibbs, C.J., & Gadjusek, D.C. (1980). Auto antibodies against axonal neurofilaments in patients with Kuru and Creutzfeld-Jakob disease. *Science, 210,* 190–193.
Steelman, L.C., & Mercy, J.A. (1983). Sex differences in the impact of the number of older and younger siblings on IQ performance. *Social Psychology Quarterly, 46*(2), 157–162.
Stubbs, E.G. (1976). Autistic children exhibit undetectable hemagglutination-inhibition antibody titres despite previous rubella vaccination. *Journal of Autism and Childhood Schizophrenia, 6,* 269–274.
Stubbs, F.G., & Crawford, M.L. (1977). Depressed lymphocyte responsiveness in autistic children. *Journal of Autism and Childhood Schizophrenia, 7,* 49–55.
Taylor, D.C. (1969). Differential rates of cerebral maturation between sexes and between hemispheres. *Lancet, II,* 140–142.

Taylor, D.C., & Ounsted, C. (1971). Biological mechanisms influencing the outcome of seizures in response to fever. *Epilepsia, 12,* 33–45.

Taylor, D.C., & Ounsted, C. (1972). The nature of gender differences explored through ontogenetic analyses of sex ratios in disease. In C. Ounsted & D.C. Taylor (Eds.), *Gender differences: Their ontogeny and significance* (pp. 215–240). London: Churchill Livingstone.

Taylor, M.A. (1969). Sex ratios of newborns: Associated with prepartum and postpartum schizophrenia. *Science, 164,* 723–724.

Taylor, P.V. (1985). Possible pathogenic effects of maternal anti-Ro (SS-A) antibody on the male fetus. *Behavior and Brain Sciences, 8,* 460–461.

Terasaki, P.I., Mickey, M.R., Yamazaki, J.N., & Vredevoe, D. (1970). Maternal-fetal incompatibility. *Transplantation, 9,* 538–543.

Thorley, J.D., Holmes, R.K., Kaplan, J.M., McCracken, G.H., & Sanford, J.P.K. (1975). Passive transfer of antibodies of maternal origin from blood to cerebrospinal fluid in infants. *Lancet, I,* 651.

Tips, R.L., Smith, G., & Meyer, D.L. (1964). Reproductive failure in families of patients with idiopathic developmental retardation. *Pediatrics, 33,* 100–105.

Toivanen, P., & Hirvonen, T. (1970a). Sex ratio of newborns: Preponderance of males in toxemia of pregnancy. *Science, 170,* 187–188.

Toivanen, P., & Hirvonen, T. (1970b). Placental weight in human foeto-maternal incompatibility. *Clinical and Experimental Immunology, 7,* 533–539.

Trites, R.L., Dugas, E., Lynch, G., & Gerguson, H.B. (1979). Prevalence of hyperactivity. *Journal of Pediatric Psychology, 4,* 179–188.

Tsai, L.Y., & Beisler, J.M. (1983). The development of sex differences in infantile autism. *British Journal of Psychiatry, 142,* 373–378.

Tsai, L., Stewart, M.A., & August, G. (1981). Implications of sex difference in the familial transmission of infantile autism. *Journal of Autism and Developmental Disorders, 11*(2), 165–173.

Vernier, M.C. (1975). Sex-differential placentation. *Biology of the Neonate, 26,* 76–87.

Vessey, M.P. (1972). Gender differences in the epidemiology of non-neurologic disease. In C. Ounsted & D.C. Taylor (Eds.), *Gender differences: Their ontogeny and significance* (pp. 203–213). London: Churchill Livingstone.

Wachtel, S.S., Koo, G.C., & Boyse, E.A. (1975). Evolutionary conservation of H-Y (male) antigen. *Nature, 254,* 270–272.

Waldrop, M.F., & Bell, R.D. (1966). Effects of family size and density on newborn characteristics. *American Journal of Orthopsychology, 36,* 544–550.

Wallace, S.J. (1974). The reproductive efficiency of parents whose children convulse when febrile. *Developmental Medicine and Child Neurology, 16,* 465–474.

Warburton, D., & Naylor, F. (1971). The effect of parity on placental weight and birth weight: An immunological phenomenon. *American Journal of Human Genetics, 23,* 41–54.

Weinberger, D.R., Cannon-Spoor, E., Potkin, S.G., & Wyatt, R.J. (1980). Poor premorbid adjustment and CT scan abnormalities in chronic schizophrenia. *American Journal of Psychiatry, 137*(11), 1410–1413.

Weizman, A., Weizman, R., Szekely, G.A., Wijsenbeek, H., Levni, E. (1982). Abnormal immune response to brain tissue antigen in the syndrome of autism. *American Journal of Psychiatry, 139,* 1462–1465.

Williams, C.A., & Schupf, N. (1977). Antigen-antibody reactions in rat brain sites induce transient changes in drinking behavior. *Science, 196,* 328–330.

Wilson, M.G., Parmelee, A.H., & Huggins, M.H. (1963). Prenatal history of infants with birth weights of 1500 grams or less. *Journal of Pediatrics, 63,* 1140–1150.

Wing, L. (1981). Sex ratios in early childhood autism and related conditions. *Psychiatry Research, 5,* 129–137.

Wolf, V. (1981). Genetic aspects of H-Y antigen. *Human Genetics, 58,* 25–28.

Wolin, S.L., & Steitz, J.A. (1984). The Ro small eytoplasmic ribonucleoproteins: Identification of the antigenic protein and its building site on the Ro RNAS. *Proceedings of the National Academy of Science of the USA, 81,* 1996–2000.

Woolf, C.M. (1971). Congenital cleft lip. A genetic study of 496 propositi. *Journal of Medical Genetics, 8,* 65–84.

Wyshak, G. (1969). Intervals between births in families containing one set of twins. *Journal of the Biological Sciences* , *1*, 337.
Zajonc, R.B. (1976). Family configuration and intelligence. *Science, 192*, 227–236.
Zajonc, R.B. (1983). Validating the confluence model. *Psychological Bulletin, 93*, 457–480.
Zerssen, D.V., & Weyerer, S. (1982). Sex differences in rates of mental disorders. *International Journal of Mental Health, 11*, 9–45.

The Neurobehavioral Effects of Early Lead Exposure

Kim N. Dietrich,
Kathleen M. Krafft,
Rakesh Shukla,
Robert L. Bornschein,
and
Paul A. Succop
University of Cincinnati

Despite the efforts of national and local health officials within the last decade, undue exposure to environmental lead (Pb) continues to be a serious pediatric health problem. Unfortunately, children at risk for lead intoxication are also likely to be exposed to a host of various biological, social, and psychological disadvantages. The interaction of these factors with Pb exposure may determine the extent and nature of the Pb-induced deficits as well as identify potential compensatory mechanisms that protect against irreversible outcomes.

Studies of the neurobehavioral effects of low to moderate childhood Pb exposure have yielded equivocal results (Bornschein, Pearson, & Reiter, 1980). Some reviewers have concluded that such inconsistent findings reflect the retrospective/cross-sectional nature of previous investigations (i.e., poor documentation of prior lead exposure and/or behavioral development) and inadequate statistical control of biological and social covariables that may mimic or obscure the health effects of lead (Pearson & Dietrich, 1985; Rutter, 1980). It has been argued that a longitudinal design is the minimum basic requirement for the reliable estimation of toxic dose and for estimation of the relative effects of Pb exposure, which may be confounded with other potent developmental influences. A prospective methodology also presents the opportunity to assess changes over age in vulnerability to Pb and the reversibility of adverse neurobehavioral response to exposure (World Health Organization, 1977).

Acknowledgements. This research was supported by a Program Project Grant from the National Institute of Environmental Health Sciences (PO1-ES-01567), Dr. Paul B. Hammond, Principal Investigator. We are grateful to the many professionals of our staff who made significant contribution to this research: Joann Grote, Leslie Harris, Mariana Bier, Susan MacDonald, Tari Gratton, Sandra Roda, Robert Greenland, and Veronica Ratliff.

Although previous cross-sectional studies have focused on the school-age child, there is a growing concern about the acute and long-term effects of fetal and infant Pb exposure. The fetal and early postnatal periods are obviously critical to adequate central nervous system structure and function. Delays in the accumulation of cerebral cytochromes and cerebral cortical synaptogenesis have been linked to prenatal Pb exposure in animal studies (Bull, Lutkenhoff, McCarty, & Miller, 1979; McCauley, Bull, & Lutkenhoff, 1979; McCauley et al., 1982). Metabolic balance studies have shown that young animals and human infants absorb and retain a higher percentage of total ingested Pb as compared with adults (Ziegler, Edwards, Jensen, Mahaffey, & Fomon, 1978). Moreover, the placenta is a poor physiological barrier for Pb (Angell & Lavery, 1982; Angle & McIntire, 1964). Further, Pb has known or highly suspected biological effects in infants and children, such as increased erythrocyte protoporphyrin (Hammond, Bornschein, & Succop, 1985; Piomelli, Seaman, Zullow, Curran, & Davidow, 1982) and depression of 1,25 dihydroxycholecalciferol (Mahaffey, Rosen, & Russell, 1982). One study even suggests that low level fetal Pb exposure may increase the probability of minor congenital anomalies (Needleman, Rabinowitz, Leviton, Linn, & Schoenbaum, 1984). However, an association between low level Pb exposure and more significant biological risks such as decreased birth weight, shortened gestation, Apgar score, or respiratory distress were not reported by Needleman, et. al.

The literature on early neurobehavioral effects of Pb exposure in human infants is meager. Well designed prospective studies during the last few years have only recently issued preliminary findings (Bornschein & Rabinowitz, 1985). Ernhart and her co-workers have examined the effect of fetal Pb exposure, as measured by maternal and cord blood lead levels, on the early neurobehavioral status of the neonate (Ernhart et al., 1985). Data from 132 mother-infant pairs from disadvantaged urban areas of a highly industrialized city included: maternal and cord blood lead, anthropomorphic dimensions, indices of early neurobehavioral status, and a set of covariates (maternal nutrition, illicit and licit drug use during pregnancy). While maternal and cord blood lead levels were highly correlated, only cord blood Pb levels were significantly associated with neurological soft signs (Rosenblith, 1979).

Bellinger, Needleman, Leviton, Waternaux, Rabinowitz, and Nichols (1984) have recently reported an inverse association between cord blood Pb levels and 6-month covariance-adjusted scores on the Mental Development Scale of the Bayley Scales of Infant Development (Bayley, 1969). However, postnatal blood Pb levels at 6 months were unrelated to behavioral development as measured by the Bayley Scales. The Bayley Scales yield a Mental Development Index (MDI) that at 6 months reflects the infant's attentiveness and responsiveness to stimuli, rudimentary problem solving, and display of early precursors of communicative behavior. While such developmental quotients are poor predictors of later childhood IQ, they are good contemporaneous indicators of neurological intactness (Ulvund, 1984).

The findings of a significant negative relationship between cord blood Pb (coded categorically as low, medium, and high) and MDI seems both surprising and alarming, given the apparently low levels of fetal exposure in the Bellinger et al. study. They reported mean cord blood Pb levels in the low, medium, and high groups of 1.8, 6.5, and 14.6 μg/dl, respectively. Also surprising is the fact that effects were found in a study sample that was predominantly white and middle to upper middle class, a sample at relatively low risk for developmental delay. While statistically significant, the negative parameter estimate for cord blood Pb category effect on Bayley MDI was quite small ($B = -2.89$). That is, a unit change in blood Pb category was associated with an estimated deficit of only 2.89 MDI points. Nevertheless, this study suggests that, even within a low risk sample, low level fetal Pb exposure has an effect on early sensorimotor development.

Moore, Goldberg, Bushnell, Day, and Fyfe (1982) examined the relationship between maternal blood Pb concentration assessed during the first trimester of pregnancy and Bayley MDI scores and Infant Behavior Record (IBR) at 12 and 24 months (Moore & Bushnell, 1984). The IBR assesses qualitative aspects of the infant's performance during the examination. Study subjects were divided into three fetal Pb exposure groups that were matched with respect to social class. The high Pb group had prenatal blood Pb values greater than 30 μg/dl whole blood; the intermediate, between 10 and 30 μg/dl; and the lowest group, less than 10 μg/dl. A stepwise regression analysis showed that birth weight, a composite measure of home environment, and socioeconomic class of the father constituted the best set of predictors for Bayley MDI at 12 and 24 months. The possibility that birth weight might be a mediating variable between prenatal Pb exposure and sensorimotor deficit was explored by removing it from the regression model. Despite this change in the regression model, Pb was not found to be a significant predictor of either 12 or 24 month MDI. In addition, correlations between IBR ratings and a composite index of Pb exposure (maternal blood Pb, home tapwater Pb, and pica at year 1 and 2) were all zero order.

In another study, Ernhart (in press) found a statistically significant negative correlation between concurrent blood Pb level and Bayley MDI at 2 years. However, after race, sex, age, parent education, maternal IQ, family authoritarian ideology, and home environment assessments were entered into regression models before Pb, the effect was no longer significant.

Although findings of early low level Pb effects on developmental outcome variables seem inconsistent, more thorough investigation of these relationships requires alternate strategies. First, in these preliminary analyses, the investigators apparently did not fully consider the possible interactions between fetal Pb exposure and other biological and social covariables known to influence developmental processes and vulnerability. Like other obstetrical or perinatal insults, fetal or early postnatal Pb exposure may most likely result in neurobehavioral delay or deficit when it occurs in the context of initial biological risk (e.g., low birth weight) or social disadvantage (e.g., lack of early stimulation and/or physical neglect) (Pearson & Dietrich, 1985).

The purpose of the present prospective investigation was to extend the database on the early behavioral effects of Pb exposure with more frequent assessment of Pb burden than previously attempted. In addition, we wanted to examine specifically the interaction between Pb exposure and other potent developmental influences using an explicit data-analytic strategy designed to address this issue as well as other statistical problems.

SUBJECTS

One hundred eighty-five expectant mothers residing in predesignated Pb-hazardous areas of Cincinnati, Ohio, were recruited at the time of their first visit to a prenatal clinic. The recruitment area was identified from the Cincinnati Lead Screening Registry as having a long history of including children with elevated blood Pb levels. Results of other studies with these children have shown that Pb from paint, dust, and generally poor housing stock is the major contributor to body burden (Clark, Bornschein, Succop, Que Hee, Hammond, & Peace, 1985).

Forty-two percent of the expectant mothers were recruited during the first trimester, 52% during the second, and 6% during the third. Women who were known to be drug addicted, alcoholic, or diabetic, or those who had documented neurological disorders, psychoses, or mental retardation were excluded from recruitment. The mean age of mothers at delivery was 23 years (S.D. = 5). Eighty-six percent of the mothers were single, and 85% were on public assistance.

Infants of less than 36 weeks gestation and/or 1500 grams were excluded from the investigation. In addition, recruited infants must have had an Apgar score of greater than 5 at 5 minutes and present no serious medical condition such as Down syndrome, phenylketonuria, polycythemia, or significant congenital anomaly.

Study infants had a mean birth weight of 3143 grams (S.D. = 463 grams) and mean gestational age by examination (Ballard, Novak, & Driver, 1979) of 39.5 weeks (S.D. = 1.7 weeks). Eighty-five percent of the infants were black, and 52% were male.

MATERIALS AND PROCEDURE

Assessment of Potential Confounders and Covariates

Undue Pb exposure is known to covary with a number of social and biological risks that may mimic, obscure, or otherwise interact with the effects of toxic exposure on neurobehavioral development (Hunt, Hepner, & Seaton, 1982; Milar, Schroeder, Mushak, Dolcourt, & Grant, 1980; Stark, Quah, Meigs, & Delouise, 1982). Therefore, a significant amount of biological and social background data were collected on all subjects. These measures are summarized in Table 1.

Nine potential covariates and/or confounders were chosen *a priori* based on their theoretical and/or known empirical relationship with both the target independent variable (Pb exposure) and/or target dependent variable (sensorimotor development). These were: (a) obstetrical complica-

TABLE 1

Arithmetic Means, Standard Deviations, and Low-High Values of Blood Lead Levels, Bayley Scales, and Covariables

VARIABLE	MEAN	STANDARD DEVIATION	LOW	HIGH
6 mo. Bayley Scales				
MDI	109.4	16.5	66	150
PDI	108.9	15.3	67	143
Blood Lead (μg/dl)				
Prenatal	8.3	3.8	1.0	27.0
10 day	4.9	3.3	1.0	24.0
3 mo.	6.3	3.8	1.0	22.0
6 mo.	8.1	5.2	1.0	36.0
Covariables+				
Obstetrical complications	82.4	6.0	68	95
Postnatal complications	94.1	10.0	30	100
Total iron binding capacity (μg/dl)	342.0	63.5	171	612
Birth weight (gms)	3143.2	463.1	1814	4394
Gestational age (weeks)	39.5	1.7	35	43
HOME	31.6	4.8	20	43
SES	17.8	5.2	8	50

+Categorical covariables (race and CITAC) are described in the text.

tions; (b) postnatal complications; (c) mother's iron status during pregnancy; (d) gestational age by examination; (e) birth weight; (f) composite index of tobacco and alcohol use during pregnancy (CITAC); (g) home environment (HOME); (h) socioeconomic status (SES); and (i) race of infant (coded 0 = white, 1 = black).

Obstetrical history and pertinent perinatal data were recorded from the neonate's and mother's charts. These data were coded using the Littman-Parmelee Obstetrical and Postnatal Complications Scales (Littman & Parmelee, 1978). Possible scale scores ranged from 0 to 100, where a high score represents no complications. A composite index of tobacco and alcohol consumption (CITAC), taken from the Problem Oriented Perinatal Risk Assessment System (POPRAS) developed by Hobel (1982), was included. The CITAC was dichotomously scored with a value of 1 indicating use of tobacco and/or alcohol during pregnancy. Fifty-six percent of the mothers in our sample reported use of these substances during the prenatal period. The mother's nutritional status during pregnancy was also assessed using a measure of total iron binding capacity (TIBC). Generally TIBC values greater than 450 indicate iron deficiency (Wintrobe et al., 1981).

The socioeconomic status (SES) of the infant's family was assessed at 3 months postpartum with the Hollingshead 4-factor Index of Social Status (Hollingshead, 1975). The mean SES for our study families was 17.8 (±5.2), reflecting the large number of single parent, low income households in the sample. At 6 months, the quality of the infant's domestic environment was assessed with Caldwell and Bradley's Home Observation for Measurement of the Environment (HOME) (Caldwell & Bradley, 1985). The HOME combines interviewer's queries with direct observations to yield a total score that reflects the parent's responsivity and involvement with her infant and the extent to which the physical environment and temporal routine is safe and stimulating. Each home visit was attended by two professionally trained observers who independently scored the HOME. Interobserver reliability on the scale was 96% for this sample (sum of agreements divided by the total number of observations). The range in HOME scores indicates a wide variation in caretaking practices within our sample of lower SES families.

Assessment of Pb Exposure and Behavioral Development

Maternal blood samples were collected by venipuncture at the first prenatal visit. Forty-three percent of these samples were collected during the first trimester, while 51% and 6% were collected during the second and third trimesters, respectively. Infant blood samples were collected at

10 days postparturition (corrected for gestational age), 3 months, and 6 months postpartum. Blood was drawn by either heel stick, finger stick, or venipuncture, depending on the physical characteristics of the infant. The percentages of blood samples drawn by a method other than venipuncture were 56%, 32%, and 34% at 10 days, 3 months, and 6 months, respectively. The arithmetic means and standard deviations for prenatal (PbBPre) and postnatal blood lead values are presented in Table 1. Postnatally, mean blood Pb levels modestly increased from 4.9 μg/dl at 10 days (PbB1) to 8.1 μg/dl at 6 months (PbB6). Interindividual exposure variability was evident at all ages. Prenatal blood Pb determinations were made by anodic stripping voltammetry by Environmental Sciences Associates, Inc. All postnatal blood samples were analyzed in duplicate for Pb in our laboratory by anodic stripping voltammetry using a Model 3010 ESA instrument (Matson, Griffin, Zink, & Sapienza, 1974; Morrel & Giridhar, 1976). All prenatal and postnatal blood Pb values were corrected for hematocrit and transformed to their natural logarithm. Our analytical laboratory participates in blood lead and protoporphyrin proficiency programs as well as maintaining an in-house program of routine benchtop and blind quality control sample analyses. These quality control procedures for the analysis of blood are detailed by Bornschein et al. (1985).

A measure of cumulative Pb exposure through 6 months of age (CumPbB6) was derived from a calculation of the area under the curve of each child's blood Pb profile from 10 days to 6 months. This composite index was used to represent historical Pb exposure in assessing early sensorimotor deficits. The intercorrelations among the Pb exposure variables are presented in Table 2.

Behavioral development was assessed at 6 months with the Mental Development Index (MDI), Psychomotor Index (PDI), and Infant Behavior Record (IBR) of the Bayley Scales of Infant Development. The Bayley Scales at 6 months provide differential indicators of the infant's

TABLE 2

Intercorrelations (Pearson r) Among LN[+] Prenatal (PbBPre) and LN Postnatal (PbB1, PbB3, PbB6, CumPbB6) Indices of Pb Exposure

	PbB1	PbB3	PbB6	CumPbB6
PbBPre	+21*	+.34**	+19*	+.34**
PbB1	—	+.49**	+.07	+.72**
PbB3	—	—	+.44**	+.87**
PbB6	—	—	—	+.55**

*p≤.01
**p≤.001
+LN = Natural Log Transformed

neurological status, and reflect attentiveness and responsiveness to stimuli, motor abilities in manipulation of objects, movement, and self-support. The IBR assesses qualitative aspects of the infant's performance during the examination. The record consists of 30 items that rate the infant's social and objective orientations toward his environment as expressed in attitudes, interests, energy level, emotions, and approach-withdrawal tendencies when stimulated. The Bayley Scales were administered in the morning at an inner city health clinic by either one of two professionally trained psychometricians. Behavioral assessments were completed prior to the medical examination. Care was taken to insure that the infant was not noticeably ill, fatigued, hungry, or under medication when examined. Intertester reliability was assessed at regular intervals throughout the study and averaged .96 (Pearson r) for the Bayley MDI and PDI. In addition, at least 85% agreement was maintained for each item of the Bayley IBR.

A principal axis factor analysis (Statistical Analysis System (SAS), 1982) of the IBR data set was executed to reduce the large number of rating variables to a few meaningful behavioral factors. A predetermined eigenvalue of 1.0 was used as the cutoff for factor extraction. Two factors were retained with eigenvalues greater than or equal to 1.0. Factor scores were based on all IBR items. AT 6 months the IBR factors were: (a) Attention/Motor Maturity and (b) Positive Mood.

Although some infants in the study scored poorly on the Bayley Scales (e.g., MDI or PDI $\leq$ 80), the vast majority presented a normal to superior pattern of early sensorimotor development, as shown in Table 1. In the U.S. population, the Bayley MDI has an estimated standarized mean of 100 and standard deviation of 16. In this sample, the mean MDI at 6 months was 109. We attribute these higher mean developmental quotients to the large number of black infants in the study. Several investigations have shown that, as a population, African and American black infants display a faster rate of motor and sensorimotor development during the first year when compared with European and North American white infants (Freedman, 1974; Scarr, 1983), although disagreement exists as to the underlying causes of this phenomenon (Super, 1976; Warren, 1972). As indicated later in this paper, these racial differences in developmental rate may plan an important role in the differential vulnerability of infants to the early adverse neurobehavioral effects of low level Pb intoxication.

DATA ANALYSIS

Controversy regarding data analysis has been at the core of recent critical commentary on published studies of the neurobehavioral effects of Pb on children (Environmental Protection Agency, 1983). Therefore, the ratonale behind the data analytic strategies used in such studies should be presented in some detail.

As previously indicated, undue Pb exposure in the United States is primarily a pediatric disease of the lower social classes who reside in urban areas (Mahaffey, Annest, Roberts, & Murphy, 1982). Lead is ubiquitous in our concentrated urban centers where there exists older deteriorated housing stock, heavy automobile traffic, and industrial sources of pollution. Undue Pb exposure in inner city children should be regarded as part of a complex of *pediatric social illnesses* in that it most often occurs in conjunction with low family income, inadequate caretaking, and few cognitive developmental resources (Hunt et al., 1982; Milar et al., 1980). Indeed, poorer caretaking practices have been shown to be a significant factor in the etiology of Pb intoxication when Pb is present in the physical environment (Dietrich et al., 1985).

The co-occurence of toxic exposure and social disadvantage in a behavioral study of the effects of Pb exposure creates a major challenge for data analyses. The independent impact of Pb exposure on developmental status and the interaction of Pb with covariables that may influence the vulnerability of infants to the neurobehavioral effects of toxic exposure (e.g., perinatal status, home environment, nutrition) must be estimated.

The list of candidate covariables is potentially enormous. For this reason, there should be solid theoretical and empirical grounds for including potential covariables and covariable by exposure variable interaction terms in regression models (Bentler, 1978; Kleinbaum, Kupper, & Morgenstern, 1982). Machine searches for potential covariables typically result in the placement of a relatively large number of independent variables in the regression model to "compete" with Pb for portions of variance in the dependent variable. This practice may present problems for data analysis because of loss of degrees of freedom when sample size is small relative to the number of covariables, inevitable collinearity among related covariables, and the potentially subtle, but not necessarily trivial, nature of the health effects of low level toxicant exposure. The net result of such a dubious procedure is a loss of statistical power and higher probability of *Type II* error—that is, incorrectly failing to reject the null hypothesis (Kleinbaum & Muller, in press). Because so many children are still exposed to Pb in the United States, *Type II* error in the evaluation of a health effect is as undesirable as *Type I* error incorrectly rejecting the null hypothesis).

The data analytic strategy outlined and utilized in this report was designed to decrease the probability of occurrence of both *Type I* and *Type II* error in the evaluation of the neurobehavioral health effects of fetal and early postnatal Pb exposure. It is appropriate for estimating the independent and interactive effects of levels of early Pb exposure measured repeatedly over time on a group of neurobehavioral outcome variables assessed at a single point in time. Each step in this data analysis strategy is outlined in Figure 1.

Data examination begins with *a priori* selection of potential *confounders* (those covariables likely to be related to both blood Pb and Bayley outcomes) and *covariates* (those covariables likely to be related to Bayley outcomes only). It is important to stress that initial selection of potential confounders and covariates is based on child development theory and a large body of previous empirical research.

In the second step, a *disease-primary trait* correlation matrix composed of candidate covariables is generated. Confounders and covariates are determined through examination of their bivariate correlations with independent and dependent variables, using a higher than standard critical p value for significance ($p \leq .10$) as recommended by Dales and Ury (1978). To assess multicollinearity among confounders, their relationship with both blood Pb level and Bayley outcomes is evaluated with hierarchical multiple regression analyses. Confounders are ordered in the hierarchical regression model based upon the value of their simple bivariate correlations in the original disease trait matrix. Confounders with higher r values enter the model first. Those confounders remaining significant within a particular blood Pb/Bayley outcome model at a p value less or equal to 0.10 are included in all further analyses of the blood Pb/ behavior relationship. Those confounders that do not remain are redesignated as *covariate-confounders* because thay are still bivariately associated with Bayley variables. These covariate-confounders are tested in the appropriate regression models in the next to last step (6). If significant, they are retained in the last step to increase the precision of parameter estimates (Kleinbaum & Muller, in press), but are not included in intermediate steps (4–5) to prevent overparameterization of regression models.

In steps 4 through 7, multivariate multiple regression (SAS, 1982) analyses are conducted to evaluate each blood Pb variable/Bayley outcome variable relationship with unique and specific confounders, covariates, and interaction terms in the regression models. To avoid overparameterization and enhance interpretation of parameter estimates, confounders and confounder interaction terms are tested first, followed by covariates and covariate interaction terms, and finally the covariate-confounders. After achieving a final unique model for each PbB variable, the parameter estimates for independent variables and particular Bayley outcomes (MDI, PDI, and IBR factors) are inspected in a univariate multiple regression analysis to determine which neurobehavioral variables were specifically affected by Pb and by other independent variables in the model.

Using this statistical approach, the probability of *Type II* error is

(1)
VARIABLE SELECTION

Initial selection of potential confounders and covariates based on theoretical and empirical studies of child development

---

xi . . . j potential
confounders and covariates

(2)
PRETESTING COVARIABLES

Generation of disease-primary trait covariance matrix composed of candidate covariables and subsequent classification as *confounder* if $p \leq .10$ for PbB *and* Bayley, or *covariate* if $p \leq .10$ for Bayley only.

---

xi . . . j confounders
xi . . . j covariates

(3)
PRETESTING CONFOUNDERS

Hierarchical multiple regression with confounders ordered on the basis of their bivariate correlations with Bayley *and* PbB is executed. Multicollinearity among confounders is controlled by retaining only those with $p \leq .10$ for a particular, unique PbB-BSID variables model.

---

xi . . . j confounders

(4)
CONFOUNDERS IN MODEL

Multivariate multiple regression test of each PbB variable relationship with set of Bayley variables in unique models with confounders and confounder by PbB interactions.

PbB (Age at collection of sample)
Confounders
Confounders × PbB

(Those confounders which are dropped are redesignated as "covariate-confounders" since they are still bivariately associated with Bayley variables. They will enter the regression models at the final steps to increase precision of parameter estimates.)

(5)
COVARIATES IN MODEL

Multivariate multiple regression test of each PbB variable relationship with set of Bayley variables in unique models with covariates, covariate by PbB interactions, confounders, and significant ($p \leq .10$) confounder by PbB interactions.

PbB (Age at collection of sample)
Confounders
Confounders × PbB ($p \leq .10$)
Covariates
Covariates × PbB

(6)
COVARIATE-CONFOUNDERS
IN MODEL

Multivariate multiple regression test of each PbB variable relationship with set of Bayley variables in unique models which include significant covariates ($p \leq .10$), significant covariate by PbB interactions ($p \leq .10$), confounders, significant confounder by PbB interactions ($p \leq .10$), and covariate-confounders.

PbB (Age at collection of sample)
Confounders
Confounders × PbB ($p \leq .10$)
Covariates ($p \leq .10$)
Covariates × PbB ($p \leq .10$)
Covariate-Confounders

(7)
FINAL UNIQUE MULTIVARIATE
MODELS

Multivariate model for each unique PbB relationship with Bayley variable set which includes confounders, significant covariates ($p \leq .05$), all significant interactions ($p \leq .05$), and significant covariate-confounders ($p \leq .05$).

PbB (Age at collection of sample)
Confounders
Confounders × PbB ($p < .05$)
Covariates ($p \leq .05$)
Covariates × PbB ($p \leq .05$)
Covariate-Confounders ($p \leq .05$)

(After achieving a final unique model for each PbB variable, the parameter estimates for individual Bayley outcomes (MDI, PDI, IBR factors) are inspected in a univariate multiple regression analysis to determine which infant neurobehavioral variables were specifically affected by Pb exposure and other independent variables in the model.)

FIGURE 1: Flow chart for general data analytic strategy used to assess the independent and/or interactive effects of fetal and early postnatal Pb exposure on infant neurodevelopmental status at 6 months.

reduced by (a) rational, *a priori* selection of covariables; (b) pretesting for confounding potential; (c) independent testing of multivariate models containing each blood Pb variable and confounders and covariates respectively; and (d) use of higher than standard critical p values for independent variable parameters until the final step. The probability of *Type I* error is reduced by (a) use of multivariate multiple regression, which considers all outcome variables collectively in the test of linear relationships, and (b) the presence of bona fide confounders in each unique model at *every* stage of hypothesis testing regardless of p value.

RESULTS

The multivariate test of a main effect for toxic exposure was statistically significant for PbB3 only (Wilks'Λ = 0.9422, $F(4,175) = 2.66$, $p < .02$). The only statistically significant multivariate interactions were those of PbB by race. There was a significant PbB3 by race interaction (Wilks'Λ = 0.9469, $F(4,175) = 2.44$, $p < .05$), and a significant CumPbB6 by race interaction (Wilks' Λ = 0.9396, $F(4,175) = 2.66$, $p < .03$). Thus, the multivariate multiple regression analyses revealed statistically significant neurobehavioral effects for the PbB3 and CumPbB6 variables only.

Table 3 presents the univariate multiple regression results for PbB3 and Bayley outcomes where a significant Pb effect was found for MDI, PDI, and the IBR Factor of Attention/Motor Maturity. In addition, a significant PbB3 by race interaction was found for MDI, PDI, and Attention/Motor Maturity.

Because the presence of a strong PbB3 by race interaction makes the parameter estimates for the PbB3 main effects uninterpretable when considered alone, the present model was reanalyzed without the interaction term. As expected, the multivariate test for the PbB3 main effect was no longer significant with exclusion of the PbB3 by race interaction (Wilks'Λ = 0.9647, $F(4,176) = 1.61$, N.S.). These results suggest that the PbB3 effect was contained in only one of the two racial subsamples.

To ascertain the nature of the PbB3 by race interaction on Bayley outcomes, separate bivariate Pearson correlations between PbB3 and neurobehavioral outcomes were obtained for black and white infants. Table 4 shows that the PbB3 effect was entirely contained in the smaller, yet highly influential subsample of white infants in the study.

Table 5 presents the univariate multiple regression results for CumPbB6 and Bayley outcomes. There was a significant main effect for CumPbB6 on MDI and PDI. A significant PbB by race interaction was also found for MDI, PDI, and the IBR Factors of Attention/Motor Maturity and Positive Mood.

TABLE 3

Univariate Multiple Regression Analysis of LN PbB at 3 Months and BSID Outcome Variables (N = 185)

BSID VARIABLE	INDEPENDENT VARIABLES	PARAMETER ESTIMATE	S.E.	p
MDI6	PbB3	−12.113	4.727	.01
$R^2 = .20$	SES	−0.206	0.222	.35
	Race	−17.573	9.457	.06
	PbB3 × race	11.859	5.075	.02
	Birth weight	0.011	0.002	.0001
	Gestational age	1.617	0.689	.02
PD16	PbB3	−13.248	4.250	.002
$R^2 = .25$	SES	−0.443	0.200	.03
	Race	−18.654	8.502	.03
	PbB3 × race	13.742	4.562	.003
	Birth weight	0.007	0.002	.003
	Gestational age	2.634	0.620	.0001
Attention/	PbB3	−0.570	0.260	.03
Motor Maturity	SES	−0.013	0.012	.28
$R^2 = .22$	Race	−1.173	0.521	.02
	PbB3 × race	0.730	0.279	.009
	Birth weight	0.0006	0.0001	.0001
	Gestational age	0.123	0.038	.001
Positive Mood	PbB3	−0.496	0.280	.08
$R^2 = .06$	SES	0.014	0.013	.27
	Race	−0.612	0.558	.27
	PbB3 × race	0.546	0.299	.07
	Birth weight	0.0002	0.00015	.19
	Gestational age	0.014	0.041	.74

TABLE 4

Bivariate Pearson Product-Moment Correlations Between 3 Months PbB and Bayley Outcomes for Black and White Infants

	WHITE INFANTS (N = 27)	BLACK INFANTS (N = 158)
MDI	−.52**	−.04
PDI	−.55**	+.01
Attention/Motor Maturity	−.45*	+.07

*p<.05
**p<.01

Examination of the CumPbB6 by race interaction on MDI, PDI, and the Attention/Motor Maturity and Positive Mood Factors yields similar results. Table 6 shows that the inverse relationship between CumPbB6 and Bayley outcomes of MDI, PDI, and the IBR Factor of Attention/Motor Maturity was entirely contained in the white subsample. It is important to point out, however, that CumPbB6 and PbB3 were highly correlated (r = +.87, p

TABLE 5

Univariate Multiple Regression Analysis of LN Cumulative Postnatal PbB (CumPbB) at 6 Months and Bayley Outcome Variables (N = 185)

BSID VARIABLE	INDEPENDENT VARIABLES	PARAMETER ESTIMATE	S.E.	p
MDI	CumPbB	−2.069	1.014	.04
$R^2 = .19$	SES	−0.167	0.222	.45
	Race	−20.275	11.698	.08
	CumPbB × race	2.285	1.079	.04
	Birth weight	0.012	0.003	.0001
	Gestational age	1.537	0.694	.03
PDI	CumPbB	−2.117	0.916	.02
$R^2 = .23$	SES	−0.385	0.201	.05
	Race	−20.841	10.564	.05
	CumPbB × race	2.547	0.874	.009
	Birth weight	0.007	0.002	.001
	Gestational age	2.576	0.626	.0001
Positive Mood	CumPbB	−0.111	0.059	.06
$R^2 = .08$	SES	0.017	0.013	.20
	Race	−1.141	0.684	.10
	Cum PbB × race	0.143	0.063	.02
	Birth weight	0.0002	0.0001	.13
	Gestational age	0.012	0.040	.78
Attention/ Motor Maturity	CumPbB	−0.092	0.056	.11
	SES	−0.115	0.012	.35
$R^2 = .22$	Race	−1.268	0.642	.05
	CumPbB × race	−0.133	0.059	.03
	Birth weight	0.0006	0.0001	.0001
	Gestational age	0.120	0.380	.0002

TABLE 6

Bivariate Pearson Product-Moment Correlations Between Cumulative Postnatal PbB at 6 Months and BSID Outcomes for Black and White Infants

	WHITE INFANTS (N = 27)	BLACK INFANTS (N = 158)
MDI	−.41*	−.01
PDI	−.42*	+.05
Attention/Motor Maturity	−.34	+.09
Positive Mood	−.40*	+.07

*p<.05

< .001). Therefore, it is likely that the CumPbB6 by race interaction was largely attributable to the contribution of 3-month PbB levels to variance in the cumulative PbB variable.

To summarize results of the multivariate analyses, low blood Pb levels at 3 months were associated with neurobehavioral deficits in white infants at 6 months of age. However, in these multivariate analyses, no index of either fetal or postnatal Pb exposure was inversely associated with developmental deficits in black infants.

Although little is known about Pb metabolism in the human fetus, it is probable that a major portion of PbB3 level is the result of resorption and equilibration of Pb laid down in bone during fetal development (Barltrop, 1969; Buchet, Roels, Hubermont, & Lauwerys, 1978). In the present investigation, support for this contention comes from the fact that early postnatal PbB was significantly correlated with prenatal (maternal) PbB (see Table 2).

This raises the important question of why neither PbBPre nor PbB1 was related to neurobehavioral status in the multivariate analyses, as these PbB assessments should also reflect primarily prenatal exposure.

It is important to point out that the statistical analyses presented above cannot adequately address the issue of whether the effects of fetal exposure on behavioral development may be indirect—that is, mediated through some other, developmentally related, biological health effect. For example, interpretive difficulties may arise when prenatal status variables are treated as confounders. Birth weight and gestational age are almost invariably entered into regression models as confounders or control variables in Pb studies. This is appropriate when interest is limited to the independent/direct or interactive effects of Pb. However, Pb exposure is a continuous environmental factor during much of the fetal period and may affect perinatal status variables such as birth weight and/or gestational age. These *nonbehavioral* health outcomes may mediate the posited relationship between developmental Pb exposure and neurobehavioral outcome. The failure to find a neurobehavioral effect for PbBPre and PbB1 suggests only that no direct effects exist; it does not preclude the possibility of mediation. Provisional support for such a developmental model comes from the fact that birth weight, gestational age, MDI, and PDI were all negatively correlated with PbBPre and PbB1 in the initial disease trait matrix. Table 7 presents the intercorrelations among these variables. For the present analysis, the most biologically significant relationship is the correlation among PbBPre, PbB1, and birth weight and gestational age. Because both birth weight and gestational age have been shown to be positively associated with early sensorimotor development in the present study and in many others (e.g., Hardy, Drage, & Jackson, 1979; Lipper, Lee, Gartner, & Grellong, 1981), fetal exposure may be indirectly related to poorer neurobehavioral status at 6 months through its effects on these perinatal status factors.

Until recently, adequate statistical techniques to estimate such indirect effects in longitudinal studies of development have not been available. Now, many of the undesirable statistical properties of path analysis and

TABLE 7

Correlations Between PbBPre, PbB1, and Perinatal and Developmental Outcomes

	PbBPre	PbB1
Birth weight	−.29**	−.14*
Gestational age	−.17*	−.08
MDI	−.13	−.13
PDI	−.16*	−.08

*$p<.05$
**$p<.001$

crosspanel correlation analysis have been solved by the method known as *structural equations* (Bentler, 1980; Seifer & Sameroff, 1982; Vinod & Ullah, 1981). Structural equation modelling may be used to test a set of specific causal hypotheses against a set of observed data (usually a covariance matrix of observed relations among the variables specified in the model).

Figure 2 shows two structural models (composed of variables in the final unique multivariate models for PbBPre and PbB1) that represent a hypothesis concerning the indirect effect of fetal Pb exposure on MDI and/or PDI. Fetal Pb exposure is posited to have an indirect effect on neurobehavioral status at 6 months through either birth weight (A) or gestational age (B). Based on previous work, the CITAC from the POPRAS is hypothesized to have a direct effect on fetal Pb (Ernhart, Wolf, Sokol, Brittenham, & Erhard, 1985; Rabinowitz & Needleman, 1984) and birth weight (Niswander & Gordon, 1972). Direct effects for fetal Pb and CITAC on sensorimotor development are also posited in the structural models.

Results of the structural equation analyses (SAS, 1982) for PbBPre and PbB1 are presented in Figure 3. In (A), all pathways were significant at the .05 level (one-tail t-test), with the exception of the direct pathways between CITAC, PbBPre, and Bayley outcomes of MDI and PDI. Significant pathways included the two that indicate an indirect effect of PbBPre on MDI and PDI through birth weight. In (B), the pathway between CITAC and gestational age was nonsignificant. However, the two pathways indicating indirect effects of PbBPre on MDI and PDI through gestational age were statistically significant at the .05 level. Finally, (C) and (D) illustrate that structural equation analyses of the PbB1 variable produced very similar but weaker relationships among hypothesized pathways as evidenced by the lower standardized partial regression coefficients.

Birthweight and gestational age are biologically related indices of perinatal health. Therefore, their independent treatment in these structural models may not always be appropriate. In a final structural

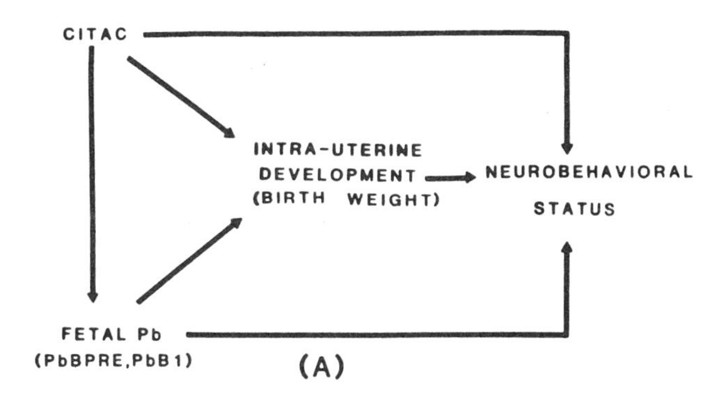

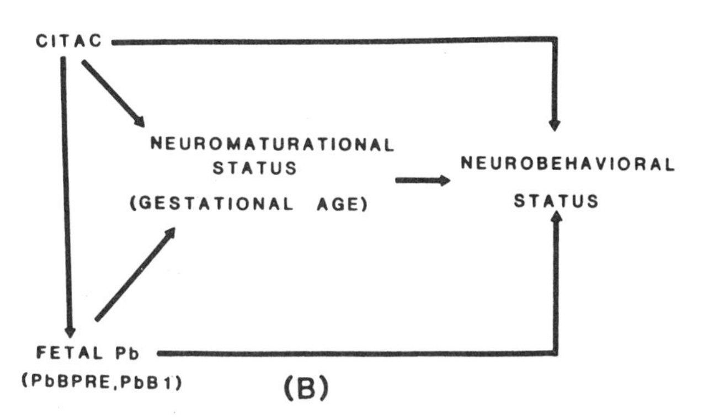

FIGURE 2. Structural Equation Models for hypothesized pathways between fetal Pb exposure, perinatal outcomes, and sensorimotor status at 6 months.

analysis, the hypothesis that fetal Pb exposure (PbBPre) influences birth weight through gestational age was explored. Figure 4 presents the results of this analysis. All pathways were statistically significant at the .05 level, with the exception of the direct paths between PbBPre, CITAC, and Bayley outcomes. While there is some evidence for an indirect effect of PbBPre on birth weight through gestational age, PbBPre (in natural log units) still made substantial independent contributions to birth weight (B = −179.5 gm) and gestational age (B = −0.6 weeks).

In summary, these structural analyses suggest that the exposure of fetuses to low levels of Pb may produce neurobehavioral deficits in young infants through lower birth weight and/or shorter gestation. Further, these effects do not seem to be limited to a small racial subsample, as was the case in the multivariate analyses for PbB3. Race was not a confounder or

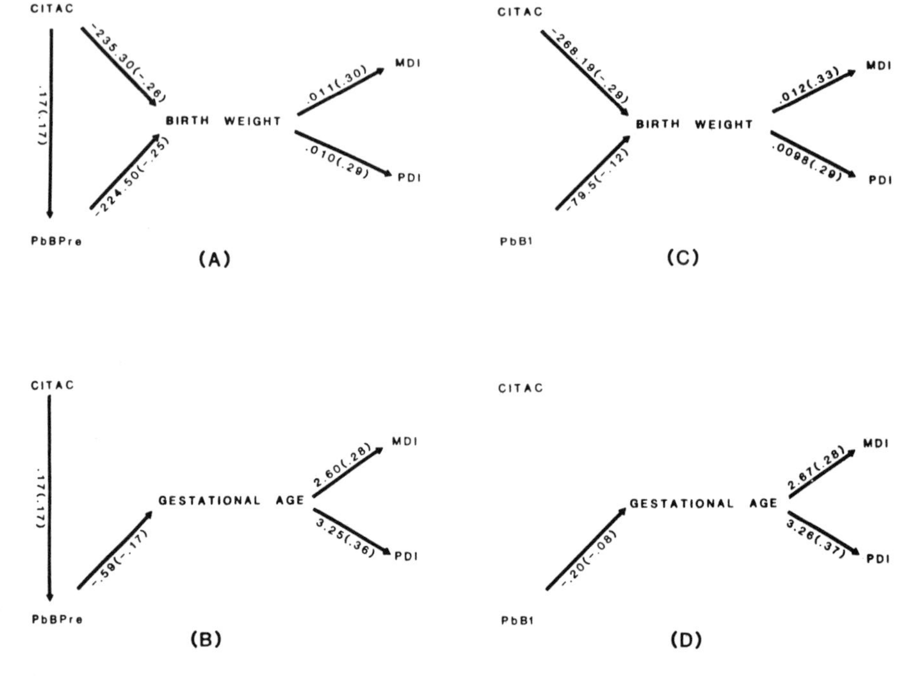

FIGURE 3. Structural Equation Analyses results for hypothesized paths among PbBPre, PbB1, Perinatal Factors, and MDI and PDI. Standardized regression coefficients in parentheses.

covariate in the final multivariate models for PbBPre or PbB1, and therefore was not directly evaluated in these structural analyses.

The lack of an inverse relationship between PbB6 and Bayley outcomes also warrants further examination. Although PbB6 was not significantly related to neurobehavioral status in the multivariate multiple regression analyses, examination of the univariate multiple regression results reveals *positive* parameter estimates for PbB6 on both MDI and PDI. For PDI, the paramater estimate for PbB6 was statistically significant ($B=4.38$, $p<.01$).

The finding of a positive relationship between PbB6 and Bayley outcomes contradicts the hypothesis of an adverse health effect as a result of postnatal Pb exposure. Further, it contradicts the finding of negative relationships between measures of fetal exposure and neurobehavioral outcome reported above. However, it should be recognized that both exposure and behavior were assessed in an organism (the human infant) whose biobehavioral organization is rapidly changing. It could be argued

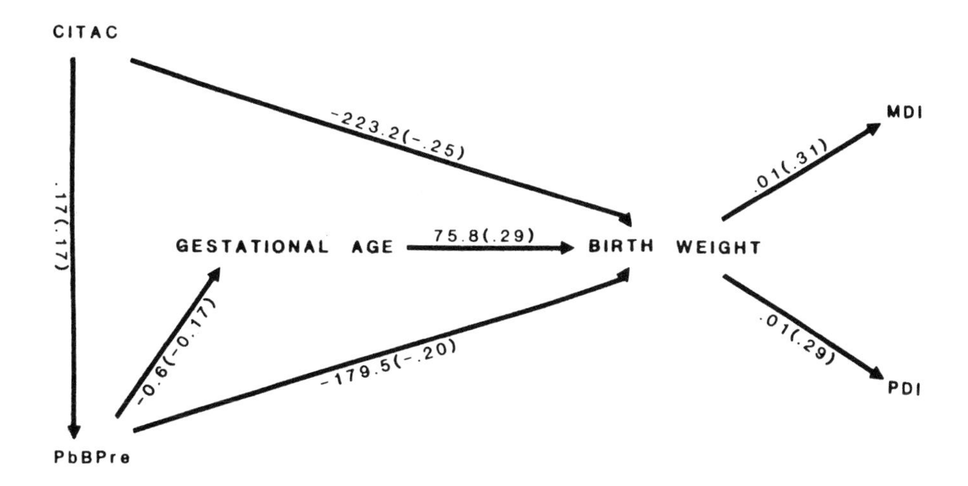

FIGURE 4. Structural Equation Analyses for hypothesized paths among PbBPre, Perinatal Factors (incorporating both Birth Weight and Gestational Age), and MDI and PDI.

that with the emergence of coordinated hand-to-mouth behavior and prewalking progression after 3 months, low level Pb exposure and the rate of early neurobehavioral development will, for a time, have a positive covariance among samples of infants living in inadequate housing where dust and soils are the major sources of Pb exposure. That is, those infants between 3 and 6 months of age who develop these behaviors first will be those more likely to access environmental sources of Pb in dust, soils, and paint. Therefore, behavioral change and toxicant exposure stand in a dynamic relationship to one another. The direction of this relationship will most likely depend on the sources (and levels) of exposure and developmental stage of the organism.

To test this hypothesis, the relationship between the *rate of change* in PbB between 3 and 6 months (adjusted for 3 month blood Pb level) and scores on 6 month Bayley MDI and PDI was examined. As predicted, those infants who evidenced the greatest increase in PbB between 3 and 6 months tended to have higher MDI and, especially, PDI scores at 6 months ($r = +.17$, $p < .03$, and $r = +.21$, $p < .01$, respectively).

To summarize, the pattern of results obtained in this investigation indicate that while low level fetal exposure to Pb may both directly (in the case of white subjects) and indirectly (for all infants) compromise neurobehavioral status at 6 months, more precocious infants may actually display higher PbB levels when postnatally exposed to sources of Pb in their physical environment. In other words, postnatal exposure and infant behavioral development stand in a dynamic relationship to one another. Developmentally advanced infants will be exposed more frequently to environmental sources of Pb as a result of their own behavior (e.g., hand-to-mouth coordinations, crawling, and visually guided reaching).

DISCUSSION

Neuronal multiplication, dendritic branching, and synaptic development occur most rapidly during the fetal period (Dobbing & Sands, 1973). Animal studies have shown that moderate Pb exposure during fetal development can delay cerebral cortical synaptogenesis and interfere with energy metabolism in the brain (McCauley et al., 1979; McCauley et al., 1982). Therefore, it might be expected that low levels of Pb exposure in the human fetus would result in early neurobehavioral deficits, such as those evidenced in this report.

However, evidence of a direct effect of Pb on neurobehavioral development seems to be robust only for the white infants in the study. This was a relatively small subsample, and any conclusions about the differential vulnerability of white and black infants to central nervous system effects of fetal Pb exposure should be appropriately guarded. Nevertheless, some authorities have argued that the more rapid rate of early sensorimotor development observed in samples of black infants has a genetic basis (e.g., Freedman, 1974; Scarr, 1983). One might speculate that early neurological development in black infants is slightly more canalized and therefore more resistant to minor forces that may perturb a normal course of early behavioral development (Waddington, 1967). It should be stressed, however, that this is merely speculation, a hypothesis that was not directly tested in the current study. These race-related results should be replicated across several studies before their implications can be seriously considered.

Perhaps most significant was the finding that the apparent early neurobehavioral effects of low level fetal Pb exposure (as indexed by PbB assessment from conception to 3 months postpartum) may be mediated through decreased birth weight and/or shortened gestation. There are a number of studies that have examined the effects of prenatal Pb exposure on obstetrical outcomes. Lead has been shown to affect placental metabolism in an *in vitro* study (Dawson, Cravy, Clark, & McGarity, 1969). There is also evidence that prematurity, lower birth weight, and premature rupture of membranes are associated with gravid maternal PbB of 30–40 μg/dl or greater (Fahim, Fahim, & Hall, 1976). However, evidence of poorer obstetrical outcomes at maternal PbB levels below 30 μg/dl has been largely negative (Alexander & Delves, 1981; Angell & Lavery, 1982; Needleman et al., 1984). Nevertheless, both birth weight and gestational age were inversely associated with low level fetal Pb exposure in this study and the neurobehavioral impact of prenatal exposure seems to be mediated through these perinatal health factors. To our knowledge, this is the first published study to report such a finding.

The findings of direct and mediated effects of fetal exposure on infant neurobehavioral status reaffirm the position taken in the introduction to this report, that Pb exposure remains a significant pediatric problem for inner city infants and children. These findings also generally concur with those of Bellinger, Needleman, Leviton, Waternaux, Rabinowitz, and Nichols (1984), who found a small but reliable inverse relationship between cord PbB and 6 month Bayley MDI. The question of whether these very early neurobehavioral effects persist, or are exacerbated by further Pb exposure and other risks, must await the maturation and further evaluation of the study cohort. However, while it is true that 6-month Bayley scores are rather poor predictors of later childhood IQ, developmental delays in infants may lead to unsatisfactory caretaker-child interactions during the first year, which may have lasting effects on development (Sameroff, 1978; Sameroff & Chandler, 1975).

Also of importance was the finding that postnatal toxicant exposure and neurobehavioral development stand in a dynamic relationship to one another. While fetal Pb exposure was associated with poorer neurobehavioral status at 6 months, postnatal Pb exposure after 3 months postpartum was actually associated with more rapid rates of sensorimotor development as indexed by the Bayley PDI. Infants who are somewhat more advanced in their motor development during the first year may actually have greater access to hazardous sources of Pb and other contaminants that may exist in the residential environment.

Developmental Pb exposure in our inner cities continues to be a serious and inadequately addressed public health problem. The findings of the present investigation indicate that adverse health effects may occur at levels far below those currently believed to be safe (Centers for Disease Control, 1985). Further research is needed both to replicate the findings reported here and to determine the long term effects, if any, of prenatal and postnatal Pb exposure.

The design, statistical analyses, and findings of this study also have implications for the entire field of child behavioral toxicology and teratology. In most studies of the behavioral effects of toxicants and teratogens, perinatal health factors such as birth weight and gestational age are treated as confounders or covariates. The results of this study indicate that such perinatal high status variables should also be explored as biological mediators of neurobehavioral delays. It is also noteworthy that only a prospective methodology with repeat measures of toxicant exposure that span the prenatal and postnatal periods could adequately address the issue of biological mediation of neurobehavioral deficits. Further, because the developing child acts upon and is in turn affected by his environment, toxicant exposure and neurobehavioral development are dynamically related. In early life, hand-to-mouth activity is normal and reflects advancements in eye-hand coordination. Infants exhibiting such activity seem to have had greater access to Pb in the current study, as reflected by their higher postnatal PbB levels at 6 months. The same phenomenon might be expected to occur for other residential contaminants that can be ingested in this manner (e.g., cadmium, arsenic, intestinal parasites such as toxocara canis). At later ages, however, a high level of hand-to-mouth activity is usually associated with developmental delay. Therefore, later deficits in cognitive development (which may have resulted from earlier Pb exposures) may lead to greater intake of Pb-laden substances from the environment.

These complicated relationships call for developmental models that go beyond those typically encountered in traditional neurotoxicology. Transactional developmental models such as those proposed by Sameroff and Chandler (1975) seem more appropriate when dealing with the complex, recursive organism-environment interactions that occur in development (see Pearson & Dietrich, 1985). It also follows that the statistical analytic techniques required to estimate the parameters of such dynamic models must go beyond traditional multiple or multivariate regression. The method known as *structural equations* seems to hold some promise for achieving this end. Our current research program is now focused on refining these developmental models and their allied statistical techniques toward a more complete description of this important public health problem.

REFERENCES

Alexander, F.W., & Delves, H.T. (1981). Blood lead levels during pregnancy. *International Archives of Occupational and Environmental Health, 48*, 35–39.

Angell, N.F., & Lavery, J.P. (1982). The relationship of blood lead levels to obstetric outcome. *American Journal of Obstetrics and Gynecology, 142*, 40–46.

Angle, C.R., & McIntire, M.S. (1964). Lead poisoning during pregnancy. *American Journal of Diseases of Children, 108*, 436–439.

Ballard, J.L., Novak, K.K., & Driver, M. (1979). A simplified score for assessment of fetal maturation of newly born infants. *Journal of Pediatrics, 95*, 766–774.

Barltrop, D. (1969). Transfer of lead to the human fetus. In D. Barltrop & W.L. Burland (Eds.), *Mineral metabolism in pediatrics* (pp. 135–151). Oxford: Blackwell.

Bayley, N. (1969). *Bayley scales of infant development*. New York: Psychological Corporation.

Bellinger, D.C., Needleman, H.L., Leviton, A., Waternaux, C., Rabinowitz, M.B., & Nichols, M. (1984). Early sensory-motor development and prenatal exposure to lead. *Neurobehavioral Toxicology and Teratology, 6*, 387–402.

Bentler, P.M. (1978). The interdependence of theory, methodology, and empirical data: Causal modeling as an approach to construct validation. In D.B. Kandel (Ed.),

Longitudinal research on drug use: Empirical findings and methodological issues. New York: Wiley.

Bentler, P.M. (1980). Multivariate analysis with latent variables: Causal modeling. *Annual Review of Psychology, 31*, 419–456.

Bornschein, R.L., Hammond, P.B., Dietrich, K.N., Succop, P., Krafft, K.M., Clark, S., Berger, O., Pearson, D., & Que Hee, S.S. (1985). The Cincinnati prospective study of low level lead exposure and its effects on child development. *Environmental Research, 38*, 4–18.

Bornschein, R.L., Pearson, D.T., & Reiter, L. (1980). Behavioral effects of moderate lead exposure in children and animal models: Part 1, Clinical studies. *CRC Critical Reviews in Toxicology, 8*, 43–152.

Bornschein, R.L., & Rabinowitz, M. (1985). Proceedings of the second international conference on prospective studies of lead. *Environmental Research, 38*, 1–2.

Buchet, J.P., Roels, H., Hubermont, G., & Lauwerys, R. (1978). Placental transfer of lead, mercury, cadmium, and carbon monoxide in women. *Environmental Research, 15*, 494–503.

Bull, R.J., Lutkenhoff, S.D., McCarty, G.E., & Miller, R.G. (1979). Delays in the postnatal increase of cerebral cytochrome concentrations in lead-exposed rats. *Neuropharmacology, 18*, 83–92.

Caldwell, B., & Bradley, R. (1985). *Home observation for measurement of the environment.* New York: Dorsey.

Centers for Disease Control. (1985). *Preventing lead poisoning in young children: A statement by the Centers for Disease Control.* Atlanta: U.S. Department of Health, Education, and Welfare.

Clark, C.S., Bornschein, R.L., Succop, P., Que Hee, S.S., Hammond, P.B., & Peace, B. (1985). Condition and type of housing as an indicator of potential environmental lead exposure and pediatric blood lead levels. *Environmental Research, 38*, 46–53.

Dales, L.G., & Ury, H.K. (1978). An improper use of statistical significance testing in studying covariables. *International Journal of Epidemiology, 7*, 373–375.

Dawson, E.B., Cravy, W.D., Clark, R.R., & McGanity, W.J. (1969). Effect of trace metals on placental metabolism. *American Journal of Obstetrics and Gynecology, 103*, 253–256.

Dietrich, K.N., Krafft, K.M., Pearson, D.T., Harris, L.C., Bornschein, R.L., Hammond, P.B., & Succop, P.A. (1985). Contribution of social and developmental factors to lead exposure during the first year of life. *Pediatrics, 75*, 1114–1119.

Dobbing, J., & Sands, J. (1973). Quantitative growth and development of human brain. *Archives of Diseases of Childhood, 48*, 757–767.

Environmental Protection Agency (1983). *Independent peer review of selected studies concerning neurobehavioral effects of lead exposures in nominally asymptomatic children: Official report of findings and recommendations of an interdisciplinary expert review committee* (EPA-600/8-83-028A). Washington, DC.

Ernhart, C.B., Wolf, A.W., Sokol, R.J., Brittenham, G.M., & Erhard, P. (1985). Fetal lead exposure: Antenatal factors. *Environmental Research, 38*, 54–66.

Ernhart, C.B., Wolf, A.W., Kennard, W.J., Filipovich, H.F., Sokol, R.J., & Erhard, P. (1985). Intrauterine lead exposure and the status of the neonate. In T.D. Lekkas (Ed.), *Proceedings of the 5th International Conference Heavy Metals in the Environment.* Edinburgh, UK: CEP Consultants, pp. 35–37.

Ernhart, C.B. (in press). Low level lead exposure and performance: The Bayley Scales of Infant Development at age two years. *Proceedings of Lead Environmental Health: The Current Issues.*

Fahim, M.S., Fahim, Z., & Hall, D.G. (1976). Effects of subtoxic lead levels on pregnant women in the state of Missouri. *Research Communications in Chemical Pathology and Pharmacology, 13*, 309–331.

Freedman, D.G. (1974). *An ethological perspective on human infancy.* Hillsdale, NJ: Lawrence Erlbaum Associates.

Hammond, P.B., Bornschein, R.L., & Succop, P. (1985). Dose-effect and dose-response relationship of blood lead to erythrocyte protoporphyrin in young children. *Environmental Research, 38*, 187–196.

Hardy, J.B., Drage, J.S., & Jackson, E.C. (1979). *The first year of life*. Baltimore: Johns Hopkins University Press.

Hobel, C.J., (1982). Development of POPRAS-problem-oriented perinatal risk assessment systm. In T.R. Harris and John P. Bahr (Eds.), *The use of computers in perinatal medicine*. New York: Praeger.

Hollingshead, A.B. (1975). *Four factor index of social status*. Unpublished manual. New Haven, CT.

Hunt, T.J., Hepner, R., & Seaton, K.W. (1982). Childhood lead poisoning and inadequate child care. *American Journal of Diseases of Children, 136*, 538–542.

Kleinbaum, D.G., Kupper, L.L., & Morgenstern, H. (1982). *Epidemiology research: Principles and quantitative methods*. Belmont, CA: Lifetime Learning.

Kleinbaum, D.G., & Muller, K.E. (in press). Assessing errors from statistical decision making in epidemiologic studies. *American Journal of Epidemiology*.

Lipper, E., Lee, K., Gartner, L., & Grellong, B. (1981). Determinants of neurobehavioral outcome in low-birth-weight infants. *Pediatrics, 67*, 502–505.

Littman, B., & Parmelee, A.H. (1978). Medical correlates of infant development. *Pediatrics, 61*, 470–474.

Mahaffey, K.R., Annest, J.L., Roberts, J., & Murphy, R.S. (1982). National estimates of blood lead levels: United States 1976–1980: Association with selected demographic and socioeconomic factors. *New England Journal of Medicine, 307*, 573–579.

Mahaffey, K.R., Rosen, J.F., & Russell, W.C. (1982). Association between age, blood lead concentration, and serum 1,25 dihydroxycholecalciferol levels in children. *American Journal of Clinical Nutrition, 35*, 1327–1331.

Matson, W.R., Griffin, R.G., Zink, E.W., & Sapienza, T.J. (1974). *An on-site procedure for micro blood lead analysis incorporating centralized quality control*. Presented at the Laboratory Directors' Conference on Pediatric Lead Poisoning. Atlanta (Reprint #R-28 from ESA, Inc.).

McCauley, P.T., Bull, R.J., & Lutkenhoff, S.D. (1979). Association of alterations in energy metabolism with lead-induced delays in rat cerebral cortical development. *Neuropharmacology, 18*, 93–101.

McCauley, P.T., Bull, R.J., Tonti, A.P., Lutkenhoff, S.D., Meister, M.V., Doerger, J.V., & Stober, J.A. (1982). The effect of prenatal and postnatal lead exposure on neonatal synaptogenesis in rat cerebral cortex. *Journal of Toxicology and Environmental Health, 10*, 639–651.

Milar, C.R., Schroder, S.R., Mushak, P., Dolcourt, J.L., & Grant, L.D. (1980). Contribution of the caregiving environment to increased lead burden in children. *American Journal of Mental Deficiency, 84*, 339–344.

Moore, M.R., Goldberg, A., Bushnell, I.W.R., Day, R., & Fyfe, M. (1982). A prospective study of the neurological effects of lead in children. *Neurobehavioral Toxicology and Teratology, 4*, 739–743.

Moore, M.R., & Bushnell, I.W.R. (1984). *Lead and child development in Glasgow: Second progress report*. Paper presented at the Second International Conference on Prospective Studies of Lead. Cincinnati, OH.

Morrel, G., & Giridhar, G. (1976). Rapid micromethod for blood lead analysis by anodic stripping voltammetry. *Clinical Chemistry, 22*, 221–223.

Needleman, H.L., Rabinowitz, M., Leviton, A., Linn, S., & Schoenbaum, S. (1984). The relationship between prenatal exposure to lead and congenital anomalies. *Journal of the American Medical Association, 251*, 2956–2959.

Niswander, K.R., & Gordon, M. (1972). *The collaborative perinatal study of the National Institute of Neurological Disease and Stroke: The women and their pregnancies*. Washington, D.C.: U.S. Government Printing Office.

Pearson, D.T., & Dietrich, K.N. (1985). The behavioral toxicology and teratology of childhood: Models, methods, and implications for intervention. *Neurotoxicology, 6*(3), 165–182.

Piomelli, S., Seaman, C., Zullo, D., Curran, A., & Davidow, B. (1982). Threshold for lead damage to heme synthesis in urban children. *Proceedings of the National Academy of Sciences USA, 79*, 3335–3339.

Rabinowitz, M.B., & Needleman, H.L. (1984). Environmental, demographic, and medical factors related to cord blood lead levels. *Biological Trace Element Research, 6,* 57–67.

Rosenblith, J.F. (1979). The Graham/Rosenblith behavioral examination for newborns: Prognostic value and procedural issues. In J.D. Osofsky (Ed.), *Handbook of infant development* (pp. 216–249). New York: Wiley.

Rutter, M. (1980). Raised lead levels and impaired cognitive functioning. *Developmental Medicine and Child Neurology, 22* (Supplement No. 42).

Sameroff, A.J., & Chandler, M.J. (1975). Reproductive risk and the continuum of care-taking casualty. In F.D. Horowitz (Ed.), *Review of child development research* (Vol. 4). Chicago: University of Chicago Press.

Sameroff, A.J. (1978). Caretaking or reproductive casualty? Determinants of developmental deviancy. In F.D. Harowitz (Ed.), *Early developmental hazards: Predictors and precautions* (pp. 79–101). Boulder, CO: Westview Press.

Scarr, S. (1983). An evolutionary perspective on infant intelligence. In M. Lewis (Ed.), *Origins of intelligence: Infancy and early childhood* (2nd ed.) (pp. 191–223). New York: Plenum Press.

Seifer, R., & Sameroff, A.J. (1982). A structural equation model analysis of competence in children at risk for mental disorder. In H.A. Moss, R. Hess, & C. Swift (Eds.), *Early intervention programs for infants* (pp. 85–97). New York: Haworth Press.

Stark, A.D., Quah, R.F., Meigs, J.W., & Delouise, E.R. (1982). Relationship of sociodemographic factors to blood lead concentrations in New Haven children. *Journal of Epidemiology and Community Health, 36,* 133–139.

Statistical Analysis System (SAS): *User's guide* (1982). Cary, NC: SAS Institute, Inc.

Super, C.M. (1976). Environmental effects on motor development: The case of "African infant precocity." *Developmental Medicine and Child Neurology, 18,* 561–567.

Ulvund, S.E. (1984). Predictive validity of assessments of early cognitive competence in light of some current issues in developmental psychology. *Human Development, 27,* 76–83.

Vinod, H.D., & Ullah, A. (1981). *Recent advances in regression methods.* New York: Marcel Dekker.

Waddington, C.H. (1967). *The strategy of the genes.* London: Allen and Unwin.

Warren, N. (1972). African infant precocity. *Psychological Bulletin, 78,* 353–376.

World Health Organization. (1977). *Environmental health criteria 3.* Geneva.

Wintrobe, M.M., Lee, R.G., Boggs, D.R., Bethell, T.C., Foerster, J., Athens, J.W., & Lukens, J.N. (1981). *Clinical hematology.* Philadelphia: Lea & Febiger.

Ziegler, E.E., Edwards, B.B., Jensen, R.L., Mahaffey, K.R., & Fomon, S.J. (1978). Absorption and retention of lead by infants. *Pediatric Research, 12,* 29–34.

Psycho-Social Factors, Lead Exposure, and IQ

Stephen R. Schroeder[1]
and
Barbara Hawk[2]
University of North Carolina

The history of research on lead is instructive. The effects of lead encephalopathy on mental retardation and deficits in motor function have been known for centuries. The amount of ambient lead in the environment increased sharply with the advent of the Industrial Revolution in the nineteenth century, so that now the average blood lead level considered acceptable in a highly industrialized nation like the U.S. may be up to 30 μg/dl (U.S. Environmental Protection Agency (EPA), 1986). This is seven times as high as average blood lead levels in Nepal, an acculturated but nonindustrialized, society (Piomelli et al., 1980).

Nevertheless, concern over asymptomatic lead exposure without the signs of encephalopathy began only about 50 years ago, when the sociopolitical climate set the stage for concern about overpopulation, abuse of natural resources, and environmental pollution. Lead then became the prototype for research on many environmental pollutants. Research emphasis focused on adverse health effects, that is, lead toxicity on organ systems of the body. Experimental prospective research was perforce done primarily on laboratory animals. Human research focused on medically oriented epidemiological studies that attempted to locate sources of exposure, at-risk populations, and environmental ecological conditions that could be used to set standards for public policy. The main question addressed by this research was finding the threshold level of lead

[1] Now at the Nisonger Center, Ohio State University.

[2] Now at Chapel Hill Pediatrics P.A., North Carolina.

Acknowledgements. We wish to acknowledge NIEHS Grant #ES-01104; EPA Grant CR809992-01-9; USPHS Grant #HD-03110 to the Child Development Research Institute; MCH Project 916 to the Division for Disorders of Development and Learning, where the children were evaluated. Thanks are also due to the Department of Pediatrics, North Carolina Memorial Hospital and the Health Effects Research Laboratories of the Environmental Protection Agency for their countless examples of support and collaboration in these projects.

burden in the body that signals an unacceptable risk for retardation of cognitive and adaptive behavior, as measured by intelligence tests, and for minimal brain dysfunction (MBD), as exemplified by hyperactivity, attention deficit disorders, fine motor skills, reaction time, etc.

LEAD EXPOSURE LEVELS

A vast body of clinical, epidemiological, and experimental data has accumulated over recent decades to show that young children, particularly preschoolers, are most at risk for the adverse effects of lead (National Academy of Sciences (NAS), 1980; U.S. EPA, 1986). The basis for this risk-effect relationship has its genesis in both the physiological status of the developing child and the relationship of the child to a given exposure setting. Young children, as developing organisms, have metabolic characteristics quite distinct from the adult human and these differences are such that they augur a deleterious outcome when a general toxicant such as lead is introduced into the picture. For example, children have an incompletely developed blood-brain barrier to movement of lead to the central nervous system. Secondly, demands of rapid growth require nutrient assimilation rates that often result in deficiencies in these factors, one result of which is that lead absorption and/or retention is enhanced (Mahaffey & Michaelson, 1980; NAS, 1976; NAS, 1980; U.S. EPA, 1986).

Children are also fundamentally distinct from adults with respect to exposure status. First, children assimilate lead in food and water at a higher rate than do adults on a body-weight or surface-area basis (NAS, 1980), absorb a greater fraction of the ingested element, and retain a greater portion of the absorbed amount (Alexander, Delves, & Clayton, 1972; Ziegler, Edwards, Jensen, Mahaffey, & Fomon, 1978). Secondly, in crawling babies the ingestion of nonfood items, such as lead contaminated dust and soil, normally occurs as part of normal behavior such as mouthing activity. In older children who frequently engage in rough-and-tumble outdoor play, lead in dust or soil is transferred to their hands and to food they hold in their hands, and is thus eventually ingested. In a setting where there is significant contamination of dust and soil, this route may dominate the dietary pathways (National Academy of Sciences, 1976, 1980).

From a historical perspective, it is quite clear that the acceptable level of exposure of children to lead and our understanding of the nature of the adverse effects engendered have been undergoing constant change. With respect to exposure, concern has shifted from such evidence of internal (or systemic) exposure as blood lead values of 60 μg/dl and higher to values considerably below this. In its 1978 statement on lead poisoning in young children (U.S. Centers for Disease Control (CDC), 1978), and directed to the pediatric community, the CDC articulated various risk categories, predicated upon an initial action level of 30 μg/dl blood lead when treatment should begin. Recently, this level has been lowered again to 25 μg/dl (U.S. CDC, 1985). Similarly, the U.S. Environmental Protection Agency established an ambient air lead standard of 1.5 μg/m3 based on what the agency took to be acceptable levels of lead exposure in children, which were below the older value of 60 μg/dl.

The compelling rationale behind a rethinking of what constitutes societally acceptable levels of pediatric lead exposure hinges on a constellation of *subclinical* or more subtle effects. Of particular concern have been the effects of lead, reported at rather low exposure levels, on heme biosynthesis, erythropoiesis, and both central and peripheral nervous system functions (Moore, Meredith, & Goldberg, 1980; NAS, 1980; Needleman & Landrigan, 1981; Piomelli, Seaman, Zullow, Curran, & Davidow, 1982; U.S. EPA, 1977). It is the issue of lead neurotoxicity at low levels of exposure that is the central focus of current research.

In the update of the EPA document *Air Quality Criteria for Lead* (U.S. EPA, 1986), we reviewed 20 of the best known studies of the neurotoxic effects of low levels of lead exposure where the children did not show the symptoms of lead encephalopathy. Table 1 shows some of the weaknesses and/or inconsistencies of these studies:

1. While several studies show statistically significant effects of lead exposure on IQ test performance, the group effects are usually small, that is, less than 6 IQ points, which is near the standard error for these tests. (Clinically significant IQ effects would be nearer to 15 IQ points—at least one standard deviation.) The IQ test, like other standardized psychometric performance tests (fine motor, reaction time, perceptual-motor tasks) may be too blunt an instrument to reliably tap subtle neurobehavioral effects of moderate lead exposure.

2. Only a few studies used a standardized rating scale for hyperactivity. However, few significant effects of asymptomatic lead exposure were found. Our group also found no effect on children age 12–72 months. (Milar, Schroeder, Mushak, & Boone, 1981.)

3. Neurological examinations yielded few lead effects below 40 μg/dl. Apparently, more sensitive neurometric measures are needed. Our group (Otto, Benignus, Muller, & Barton, 1981) demonstrated significant amplitude changes in slow wave potentials of children aged 12–47 months with 6–59 μg/dl, while this effect did not appear in older children (48–75 mos.).

4. No study has evaluated children's intelligent or social behavior based on a theoretical hypothesis as to the nature of the cognitive, attentional, and perceptual-motor deficits that have often been found on IQ tests and attention deficit questionnaires.

TABLE 1

Summary of Studies on Neurobehavioral Functions of Lead-Exposed Children[a]

Reference	Population studied	N/group	Age at testing, yr (range)	Blood lead, μg/dl (range or ± S.D.)	Psychometric tests employed	Summary of results				Levels of signifi-cance[b]
Clinic-type Studies of Children with High Lead Levels										
							C	Pb		
de la Burde and	Inner city	C = 72	4.0	?[c]	IQ (Stanford-	Score:	94	89		
Choate (1972)	(Richmond, VA)	Pb = 70	4.0	58 (30–100)[d]	Binet)	% subnormal:[e]	10	25		<.05
					Fine motor		26	45		<.05
					Gross motor		7	16		N.S.
					Concept formation		10	15		N.S.
					Behavior profile		10	30		<.01
de la Burde and	Follow-up	C = 67	7–8	PbT: 112 μg/g	WISC Full Scale	Score:	90	87		
Choate (1975)	same subjects	Pb = 70	7–8	202 μg/g	IQ	% subnormal:[e]	6	24		.01
					Verbal IQ		9	18		N.S.
					Performance IQ		13	24		N.S.
					Bender-Gestalt		27	49		.01
					Reading		7	12		N.S.
					Spelling		11	16		N.S.
					Arithmetic		7	12		N.S.
					Goodenough-Harris draw test		1	13		.02
					Auditory vocal assoc.		13	31		.01
					Tactile recognition		3	15		.05
					Behavior profile		3	25		.001
Rummo (1974);	Inner city	C = 45	5.8 (4–8)	23 (±8)	McCarthy Scales:	C	Pb_1	Pb_2	Pb_3	
Rummo et al.	(Providence, RI)	$Pb_1 = 15$	5.6	61 (±7)	Gen. cognitive	93	94	88	77	<.01
(1979)		$Pb_2 = 20$	5.6	68 (±13)	Verbal	46	46	44	37	<.05
		$Pb_3 = 10$	5.3	88 (±41)	Perceptual	48	49	46	38	<.05
					Quantitative	45	44	41	35	<.01
					Memory	47	46	43	36	<.01
					Motor	52	52	50	40	<.01
					Parent ratings	8	10	10	18	<.01
					Neurologic exam	7/12 measures sig. different				
Kotok (1972)	Inner city	C = 25	2.7 (1.1–5.5)	38 (20–55)	Denver Developmental:	Norm	C	Pb		
	(New Haven, CT)	Pb = 24	2.8 (1.0–5.8)	81 (58–137)	Gross motor	1.00	1.02	1.06		N.S.
					Fine motor	1.00*	.82	.81*		*<.01
					Language	1.00*	.82	.73*		*<.01

TABLE 1

Summary of Studies on Neurobehavioral Functions of Lead-Exposed Children[a] (Continued)

Reference	Population studied	N/group	Age at testing, yr (range)	Blood lead, µg/dl (range or ± S.D.)	Psychometric tests employed	Summary of results		Levels of significance[b]
Kotok et al. (1977)	Inner city (Rochester, NY)	C = 36 Pb = 31	3.6 (1.9–5.6) 3.6 (1.7–5.4)	28 (11–40) 80 (61–200)	IQ Equivalent:	C	Pb	
					Social	126	124	>.10
					Spatial	101	92	<.10
					Spoken vocal	93	92	>.10
					Info-comprehension	96	94	>.10
					Visual attention	93	90	>.10
					Auditory memory	100	93	>.10
Smelter Area Studies								
						C	Pb	
Landrigan et al. (1975)	Smelter area (El Paso, TX)	C = 78 Pb = 46	9.3 8.3 (3.8–15.9)	<40 40–68	WISC Full Scale IQ[f]	93	89	N.S.
					WPPSI Full Scale IQ[g]	91	86	N.S.
					WISC + WPPSI Combined	93	88	N.S.
					WISC + WPPSI Subscales	C > Pb on 13/14 scales 7/14 scales sig. different		<.05
					Neurologic testing	C > Pb on 7/8 tests 1/8 tests sig. different		<.01
McNeil et al. (1975)	Smelter area (El Paso, TX)	C = 37 Pb = 101	9 9 (1.8–18)	29 (14–39) 58 (40–93)	McCarthy General	C	Pb	
					Cognitive	82	81	N.S.
					WISC-WAIS Full Scale IQ	89	87	N.S.
					Oseretsky Motor Level	101	97	N.S.
					California Personality	C > Pb, 6/10 items		<0.05
					Frostig Perceptual Quotient	100	103	N.S.
					Finger-Thumb Apposition	27	29	N.S.
						Mod.	High	
Ratcliffe (1977)	Smelter area (Manchester, UK)	Mod. Pb = 23 Hi Pb = 24	4.7 (4.1–5.6) 4.8 (4.2–5.4)	28 (18–35) 44 (36–64)	Griffiths Mental Dev.	108	102	N.S.
					Frostig Visual Perception	14.3	11.8	N.S.
					Pegboard Test			
					Dominant hand	17.5	17.3	N.S.
					Nondominant hand	19.5	19.8	N.S.

TABLE 1

Summary of Studies on Neurobehavioral Functions of Lead-Exposed Children[a] (Continued)

Reference	Population studied	N/group	Age at testing, yr (range)	Blood lead, μg/dl (range or ± S.D.)	Psychometric tests employed	Summary of results		Levels of significance[b]
						C	Pb	
Winneke, Hrdina, & Brockhaus (1982)	Smelter area (Duisberg, FRG)	C = 26	8	PbT = 2.4 ppm[h]	German WISC Full Scale	122	117	N.S.
		Pb = 26	8	PbT = 9.2 ppm	Verbal IQ	130	124	N.S.
				No PbB	Performance IQ	130	123	N.S.
					Bender Gestalt Test	17.2	19.6	<.05
					Standard Neurological Tests	2.7	7.2	N.S.
					Conners Teacher Ratings	?	?	N.S.
Perino and Ernhart (1974)*	Inner City (New York, NY)	Low Pb = 50	3–6	10–30	McCarthy Scales:	Low	Mod.	
		Mod. Pb = 30	3–6	40–70	Gen. cognitive	90	80	<.01
					Verbal	44	39	<.05
					Perceptual	44	37	<.05
					Quantitative	48	44	N.S.
					Memory	45	42	N.S.
					Motor	46	42	N.S.
Ernhart et al. (1981)*	Follow-up same subjects	Low Pb = 31	8–13	21 (±4)	McCarthy Scales:	Low	Mod.	
		Mod. Pb = 32		32 (±5)	Gen. cognitive	94	82	<.05
					Verbal	48	41	<.05
					Perceptual	43	40	N.S.
					Quantitative	43	38	N.S.
					Memory	44	39	N.S.
					Motor	49	46	<.05
					Reading tests	Not Reported		N.S.
					Conners teacher ratings	Not Reported		N.S.
					Various experimental tests	Not Reported		N.S.
General Population Studies								
Needleman et al. (1979)**	Urban (Boston, MA)	C = 100	7	PbT: <10 ppm[h]	WISC Full Scale IQ	106.6	102.1	.03
		Pb = 58	7	>20 ppm	Verbal IQ	103.9	99.3	.06
					Performance IQ	108.7	104.9	.12
					Seashore Rhythm Test	21.6	19.4	.002
					Token Test	24.8	23.6	.09
					Sentence Repetition Test	12.6	11.3	.04
					Delayed Reaction Time	C > Pb on 3/4 blocks		<.01
					Teacher Ratings	9.5	8.2	.02

TABLE 1

Summary of Studies on Neurobehavioral Functions of Lead-Exposed Children[a] (Continued)

Reference	Population studied	N/group	Age at testing, yr (range)	Blood lead, μg/dl (range or ± S.D.)	Psychometric tests employed	Summary of results	Levels of signifi-cance[b]
McBride et al.	Urban/suburban	Low Pb = >100	4,5	2–9 μg/dl	Peabody Picture	Low Mod.	
(1982)	(Sydney, Australia)	Mod. Pb = >100	4,5	19–29 g/dl	Vocab. Test	~105 ~104	N.S.
					Fine Motor Tracking	C > Pb 1/4 comparisons	<0.05
					Pegboard	~20 ~20	N.S.
					Tapping Test	~30 ~31	N.S.
					Beam Walk	~5 ~4	N.S.
					Standing Balance	C < Pb 1/4 comparisons	<0.05
					Rutter Activity Scale	~1.9 ~2.1	N.S.
						Group: 1 2 3 4	
Yule et al.	Urban	Group 1 = 34	9	8.8[j] (7–10)	WISC-R Full Scale IQ	103 103 96 96	.027
(1981)	(London, UK)	Group 2 = 48	9	11.6 (11–12)	Verbal IQ	101 101 95 94	.043
		Group 3 = 49	8 (6–12)	14.5 (13–16)	Performance IQ	106 03 98 99	.102
		Group 4 = 35	8	19.6 (17–32)	Vernon Spelling Test	104 98 92 89	.001
					Vernon Math Test	97 97 95 95	N.S.
					Neale Reading Accuracy[k]	121 110 96 89	.001
					Neale Reading Compre.[k]	117 110 95 88	.001
						Group: 1 2 3 4	
Yule et al.	Same subjects	Same	Same	Same	Needleman Teacher	1.53 1.54 2.45 2.63	.096
(1984)	in Yule et al. (1981)				Ratings	(4/11 items sig. different)	
					Conners Teacher	.26 .37	.04
					Ratings	(3/4 factors sig. at p <.05)	
					Rutter Teacher	(2/26 items sig. at p≤.05)	
					Ratings, including	(5/26 items differ at .05<p<.10)	
					"Overactivity" factor	6% 4% 20% 17%	.04
						Low High	
Yule and Lansdown	Urban	80	9	7–12	WISC-R Full Scale	107 105	N.S.
(1983); Yule	(London, UK)	82	9	13–24	Verbal IQ	104 103	N.S
et al. (1983)					Performance IQ	108 106	N.S.
					Neale Reading Accuracy	114 111	N.S.
					Neale Reading Comprehension	113 109	N.S.
					Vernon Spelling	101 99	N.S.
					Vernon Math	100 99	N.S.

TABLE 1

Summary of Studies on Neurobehavioral Functions of Lead-Exposed Children[a] (Continued)

Reference	Population studied	N/group	Age at testing, yr (range)	Blood lead, μg/dl (range or ± S.D.)	Psychometric tests employed	Summary of results			Levels of significance[b]
						Low	Med	High	
Smith et al. (1983)	Urban (London, UK)	Hi = 155	6,7	PbT ≥ 8.0	WISC-R Full Scale	107	105	105	N.S.
		Med = 103	6,7	PbT = 5–5.5	Verbal IQ	105	103	103	N.S.
		Low = 145	6,7	PbT < 2.5	Performance IQ	108	106	106	N.S.
				(All in μg/g)	Word Reading Test	45	42	40	N.S.
				$\bar{X}$ PbB = 13.1	Seashore Rhythm Test	21	20	20	N.S.
				μg/dl	Visual Sequential Memory	20	19	20	N.S.
					Sentence Memory	9	9	9	N.S.
					Shape Copying	14	14	14	N.S.
					Mathematics	16	15	15	N.S.
					Mean Visual RT (secs)	.37	.37	.39	N.S.
					Conners Teacher Ratings	11	11	13	N.S.
Harvey et al. (1983, 1984)	Urban (Birmingham, UK)	189	2.5	15.5 (6–30)	British Ability Scales	Regression F Ratio			
					Naming		<1		N.S.
					Recall		1.26		N.S.
					Comprehension		<1		N.S.
					Recognition		<1		N.S.
					IQ		<1		N.S.
					Stanford-Binet Items				
					Shapes		<1		N.S.
					Blocks		2.34		N.S.
					Beads		2.46		N.S.
					Playroom Activity		?		N.S.
Winneke et al. (1983)	Smelter area (Stolburg, FRG)	89	9.4	PbT: 6.16 ppm[h] PbB: 14.3 μg/dl	German WISC	% Variance Due to PbT			
					Full Scale IQ		−0.0		N.S.
					Verbal IQ		−0.5		N.S.
					Performance IQ		+0.6		N.S.
					Bender Gestalt Test		+2.1		<0.05
					Standard Neurological Tests		+1.2		N.S.
					Conners Teacher Ratings		0.4–1.3		N.S.
					Wiener Reaction Performance		+2.0		N.S.

TABLE 1

Summary of Studies on Neurobehavioral Functions of Lead-Exposed Children[a] (Continued)

Reference	Population studied	N/group	Age at testing, yr (range)	Blood lead, µg/dl (range or ± S.D.)	Psychometric tests employed	Summary of results	Levels of significance[b]
Winneke et al. (1984)	Smelter area (Nordenham, FRG)	122	6.5	8.2 (4.4–22.8)	German WISC	% Variance Due to Pb	
					Short form	−0.3	N.S.
					Verbal IQ	+0.3	N.S.
					Performance	−2.4	N.S.
					Bender Gestalt Test	+0.5	N.S.
					Signalled Reaction Time		
					Short	+0.1	N.S.
					Long	−0.2	N.S.
					Wiener Reaction Time		
					Easy	+4.3	<0.05
					Difficult	+11.0	<0.01

[a]Abbreviations: C = control subjects; Pb = lead-exposed subjects; N.S. = nonsignificant ($p>.05$); PbT = tooth lead; WISC = Wechsler Intelligence Scale for Children; WPPSI = Wechsler Preschool and Primary Scale of Intelligence; RT = Reaction Time. [b]Significance levels are those found after partialing out confounding covariates. [c]Urinary coproporphyrin levels were not elevated. [d]Some with positive radiologic findings, suggesting earlier exposure in excess of 40–60 µg/dl. [e]Percent of each group scoring "borderline," "suspect," "defective," or "abnormal." [f]Used for children over 5 years of age. [g]Used for children under 5 years of age. [h]Main measure was dentine lead (PbT). [i]Dentine levels not reported for statistical reasons. [j]Blood lead levels taken 9–12 months prior to testing; none above 33 µg/dl. [k]Data not corrected for age. *Reanalysis of data by Ernhart correcting for methodological problems in earlier published analyses described here mainly did not substantiate significant differences between control and Pb-exposed children indicated in last two columns to the right (see chapter text). **Reanalyses of Needleman data correcting for methodological problems in earlier published analyses confirmed significant differences between study groups indicated in last two righthand columns for WISC IQ test results (see chapter text).

5. Epidemiological studies have not followed up on these children to evaluate the cumulative clinical effects of lead exposure or reversibility upon removal of lead from his/her home environment.

6. The long-term clinical neurotoxic effects of moderate lead exposure on children's development largely remain to be investigated.

7. Epidemiological studies that have been done point to the presence of a hazard caused by lead and the need for guidelines to regulate exposure in the general population. But they are of limited help in predicting the outcome of individuals with specific deficits that vary along continuous behavioral dimensions interacting with social and developmental factors.

RESEARCH DIFFICULTIES

Biological Indices

In addition to the above, there are some general, pervasive difficulties in lead research. The first is the highly controversial issue of the best biological index of internal, or systemic, exposure to lead. A growing data base dealing with lead toxicokinetics provides some useful guides in considering a choice of exposure index.

Blood lead measurement, to the extent that it can be accurately determined in a given laboratory, is dependent for its usefulness on the nature of the exposure being sustained by the study population. Lead absorbed into the bloodstream is cleared from blood to tissues on the order of weeks or several months (Chamberlain, Heard, Little, Newton, Wells, & Wiffen, 1978; Rabinowitz, Wetherill, & Kopple, 1977). Hence, it is most useful with chronic elevated exposure and less so with episodic bouts of lead intake. Measurement of lead in an accessible, accumulating matrix such as shed dentition pushes back the exposure period to years, but this measure is by its nature retrospective (see Needleman et al., 1979). One analyzes shed dentition to ascertain whether lead exposure *occurred*, rather than *is occurring*.

Hence, while dentition analysis is more appropriate in defining aggregate exposure and its relationship to health measures, it does not provide a useful regulatory metric for monitoring lead exposure in real time or concurrent lead intake versus change in outcome measure assessment. In the absence of available methods for *in situ* measurement of lead in children during their most vulnerable stage of development, the best compromise seems to be *serial* blood lead measurements, for example, quarterly. Such serial measurements would, of course, increase the reliability of using blood lead as the exposure index because increases in chronic exposure would be ascertainable while the occurrence of episodic intake of large amounts of lead would be more likely to be captured in laboratory analysis with frequent sampling.

Exposure indicators that directly reflect a biological lesion are also of value when taken in tandem with blood lead values (CDC, 1978). At present, the indicator of most utility of this type is free erythrocyte protoporphyrin (FEP), a heme precursor whose elevation is related more to chronic than to episodic exposure.

Social Factors

The second challenge is a growing understanding of and concern over the interrelationships among social factors, lead, and child IQ.

The contribution of maternal intelligence to the child's intelligence must also be evaluated in carefully controlled studies of lead effects on intelligence. Heber (1970) found a high concordance between maternal and child intelligence. A majority of the children with IQs in the retarded range have mothers with IQs of less than 80. He also found a decline in IQ range for lower socioeconomic status (SES) children with increasing age. For mothers with IQs less than 80, the percentage of their children with IQs less than 80 increased from 20% for ages under 6 years of age to 90% for those over 13. If mothers of lead exposed children have IQs less than 80, then intellectual differences previously attributed to lead might also be explained by maternal IQ.

Most studies have attempted to control for possible covariates (Table 2) such as social class, age, maternal IQ, pica, and parents' attitude toward education, but not for the quality of the caregiving environment.

Studies examining the relationship between socioeconomic status and intelligence and academic achievement have yielded mixed results. In a meta-analysis of 200 studies relating SES to academic achievement, White (1982) found that home atmosphere correlated to a much higher degree with academic achievement than any other combination of SES indicators. The more important variables were the childrearing practices and stimulation of learning at home and school, and not parents' occupation, income, or education. In general, SES seems to be a broad but crude measure of factors such as caregiving practices, resources, etc., that may be better examined individually.

The Influence of Caregiving

The results of previous research have suggested that there might be *deficiencies in the caregiving environment* of children who evidence increased

TABLE 2

Evaluation of Control of Confounding Variables of the Twenty Major Studies on Low to Moderate Blood Lead Levels in Children

	Possible Confounding Variables Controlled (indicated by +							
	SES	Age	Pica	Blind Eval.	Home Envir.	Race	Mat. IQ	Exposure History
de la Burde & Choate (1972)	+	+		+	+	+	+	
Kotok (1972)	+	+	+			+		
Lansdown et al. (1974)								+
Perino & Ernhart (1974)	+	+				+	+	
de la Burde & Choate (1975)	+	+		+	+	+	+	
Landrigan et al. (1975)	+		+					+
McNeil et al. (1975)	+	+	+	+		+	+	
Kotok et al. (1977)	+	+	+		+	+		
Ratcliffe (1977)	+	+						+
Needleman et al. (1979)	+	+	+	+		+	+	+
Rummo et al. (1979)	+	+		+		+		+
Ernhart et al. (1981)	+	+				+	+	
Yule et al. (1981, 1984)	+	+						+
McBride et al. (1982)	+		+			+		
Winneke, Hrdina, & Brockhaus (1982)	+	+	+					
Harvey et al. (1983)	+		+			+		+
Smith et al. (1983)	+	+	+			+		+
Winneke et al. (1983)	+	+						+
Yule et al. (1983)	+	+						+
Winneke & Kraemer (1984)	+	+	+					+

lead burden (Chatterjee & Gettman, 1972; Lansdown, Sheperd, Clayton, Delves, Graham, & Turner, 1974; Millican, Lourie, & Layman, 1956; Rennert, Weiner, & Madden, 1970; Rummo, Routh, Rummo, & Brown, 1979).

Milar, Schroeder, Mushak, Dolcourt, and Grant (1980) compared two groups of children, 12–30 months of age and 31–78 months of age, showing increased lead burden with a sample of children matched for age, sex, and socioeconomic status, but showing no evidence of increased lead burden. The quality of the caregiving environment of these children was assessed with the Home Observation for Measurement of the Environment (HOME) Inventory developed by Caldwell, Heider, and Kaplan (1966). A measure of maternal intelligence was also obtained. For younger children in the sample, significant deficits in maternal IQ and quality of the caregiving environment were associated with increased lead burden. Subscales of the HOME Inventory dealing with emotional and verbal responsivity of the mother and maternal involvement with the child showed significant deficiencies in the caregiving environment of the children with increased lead burden. For older children, the HOME

Inventory also showed deficiencies in the caregiving environment with increased lead burden, but the differences were statistically not significant.

Research has only recently begun to document the powerful influences of the early caregiving environment on subsequent development of the child. Studies by Bradley and Caldwell (1976a, b) used the HOME Inventory to identify factors in the child's environment during the first two years of life that are related to mental test performance at 36 and 54 months of age. Two of the subscales of the HOME Inventory that were strongly related to later intellectual development were emotional and verbal responsivity of the mother and maternal involvement with the child. These are the two subscales identified by Milar et al. (1980) showing significant deficiencies in the environment of children with increased lead burden.

Traditionally, the interpretation of the research on lead effects in humans has been that increased lead burden directly results in deficits in cognitive functioning. However, alternative hypotheses are equally plausible. First, the results of Milar et al. (1980) suggest the possibility that deficits found in children exposed to lead may be a direct result of deficiencies in the caregiving environment and may not be related to lead at all. The research of Bradley and Caldwell (1976a, b) tends to support this conclusion.

Second, it is possible that deficiencies in the caregiving environment are responsible for increased lead burden and that the deficiencies are caused by lead. A child in an environment where lead is available would be much more likely to ingest significant amounts of lead if left unsupervised by his/her caregiver. The poor caregiving environment may be an antecedent to the lead ingestion, but the neurotoxic effects of lead may be responsible for observed deficits in cognitive functioning. This situation may be analogous to malnutrition in children. Severe malnutrition can lead to cognitive deficits (Dobbing, 1970), but Cravioto and DeLicardie (1972) have also documented that aspects of the caregiving environment may place children at risk for malnutrition.

A third hypothesis is that the caregiving environment and lead combine to affect intellectual development adversely. This would be similar to the relationship found by Werner, Honzik, and Smith (1968) between perinatal complications and later psychological development. At 20 months of age IQ differences between children with and without perinatal complications were only 5–7 points for children from a favorable social background; but for infants living in a low socioeconomic environment, the IQ differences ranged from 19–37 points. Apparently, perinatal insult and the quality of the child's environment both affected development. Similarly, even with low lead levels, we might anticipate a combined effect of SES, maternal IQ, the caretaking environment, inadequate nutrition, and lead, each of which by itself is not significant, but when combined with the others poses a cumulative risk of handicaps in the development of cognitive and adaptive behavior.

THE DEVELOPMENTAL PERSPECTIVE

The epidemiological studies presented earlier on the toxicology of lead have been very valuable for dealing with the acute effects of lead exposure, but they have been only modestly helpful in addressing its chronic effects. A developmental perspective, in addition to defining who is at risk, what is wrong, and how the disease can be corrected, also asks what the cumulative risks on functioning at a later age are within one's ecological context and how these adverse effects can be compensated for, reversed, or at least minimized.

Focusing investigative efforts on younger populations has other advantages when one considers that possible neurological insult resulting from lead takes place within a developmental context. Sameroff and Chandler (1975) pointed out that that even serious insults such as anoxia and prematurity often have transient effects. If the exposure to lead occurred many years before, a robust deficit may not still be present because of the reversibility of effects. They also pointed out that the severity of effect could be lessened by a favorable home environment. In addition, during the first two years of life, brain growth is very rapid and the brain is more vulnerable to insult (Dobbing, 1970). The possibility of differential effects of lead dependent on the age at exposure has not been carefully investigated.

The majority of children evaluated in studies investigating possible subclinical effects of lead were more than five years old. It has been documented (CDC, 1978) that children between 1 and 3 years of age are most susceptible to lead poisoning. The subsequent evaluation of children two or more years after exposure to lead makes it difficult to retrospectively determine the extent and duration of a child's lead exposure. By studying younger populations of children, the influence of uncontrolled and unknown events affecting development is reduced because of the recency of the lead exposure.

By adding the developmental perspective and recognizing the ethical limitations of doing prospective lead studies on children, it seems that lead investigators should take a lesson from related fields like nutrition. Decades of research attempts in nutrition have failed to clarify a causal relationship between malnutrition and specific psychological developmental variables in children (Read, 1982). As with malnutrition, it may be impossible to isolate the causal effects of lead independent of the social conditions in which they occur. Perhaps we should move beyond the assumption that there is a direct causal relationship between lead exposure, altered brain development, and impaired behavioral functioning and focus instead on: (a) more systematic analysis of the ways in which the child's lead exposure, social environment, and early experience interact in jointly to influence the course of his psychological development, with more precise assessment of lead exposure and behavioral development; (b) a fuller understanding of the mechanisms through which lead exposure may affect intellectual and adaptive behavior development; and (c) evaluation of the effectiveness of systematic efforts to prevent or reverse the detrimental consequences of early lead exposure.

This latter strategy has been pursued by studies that have tried to evaluate the effects of lead chelation therapy (see Rutter, 1980, for review). We took a similar strategy with a longitudinal and cross-sectional study of the intellectual, social, and neurobehavioral development of preschool children exposed to low (10–30 μg/dl) or moderate (30–60 μg/dl) blood lead levels. We asked two questions: (a) Does cross-sectional comparison show a significant interaction between age and blood lead levels, between age and type of exposure (occupational vs. nonoccupational), or between age and the important behavior covariates of lead exposure (socioeconomic status, maternal IQ, and quality of the caregiving environment); and (b) Upon regular five-year reevaluations, is there a change in these children's intellectual, social, and neurobehavioral development that can be related to current blood levels or to cumulative previous blood lead levels after removal of lead from their home environments?

GENERAL METHODOLOGY

Populations Sampled

Several sources were utilized to recruit subjects for this project. These sources included: (a) referrals from the statewide Early and Periodic Screening, Diagnosis, and Treatment (EPSDT) Program; (b) referrals from local lead screening programs in Wake, Lenoir, and New Hanover counties, and (c) direct recruitment of children from families employed or residing near lead-related industries. Direct contact, recruitment, and scheduling of subjects were done by the Patient Coordinator through local or county health departments under the aegis of the North Carolina Statewide Lead Screening Advisory Committee. A description was sent to all county health departments to inform them of the objectives and resources of the research project and to encourage referrals as new cases of elevated PbB levels are discovered. Descriptions of recruitment sources follow.

EPSDT Program

The North Carolina EPSDT Progam, implemented under Title XIX of the Social Security Act (Medicaid Law), provided general medical screening for lower income families. All Medicaid eligible familes were informed that screening is available, but participation in the EPSDT program was voluntary. Screening was performed by county health departments and local well-baby clinics. One component of the screening program was a *lead poisoning test* performed between 12 and 60 months of age. This test determined the free erythrocyte protoporphyrin (FEP) level using a hematofluorimeter and capillary blood sample (fingerprick). If the level of FEP, a measure of heme synthesis, was greater than 50 μg/dl, a venipuncture blood sample was drawn and sent to the North Carolina Division of Health Services (NCDHS) for blood lead analysis. If the PbB levels were $>$ 50 μg/dl, children were referred to appropriate medical facilities for chelation treatment to reduce PbB levels. If PbB levels were between 30 and 50 μg/dl, the county health department was instructed to send periodic blood samples to the state lab to monitor PbB levels. A home visit team was also sent to identify the source of lead and to initiate appropriate abatement procedures to eliminate the source of contamination. A flow diagram of the screening, treatment, and abatement procedures implemented in Wake County is shown in Figure 1.

NCDHS provided data from screening probes by the Environmental Epidemiology Branch for the purpose of determining the frequency of occurrence of elevated FEP/PbB cases by county during 1981 and previous years. This procedure permitted the identification of "hot spots" for study purposes and the evaluation of county compliance with the EPSDT Pb screening program. A list of potential subjects for the proposed studies was also obtained in this manner. Available data from NCDHS records included birthdates, sex, race, county, FEP, PbB, and the date that the blood sample was drawn from each child. Contact with individual families was arranged and coordinated through county or local health agencies participating in the EPSDT Program. NCDHS has perfomed about 10,000 PbB analyses during each of the past five years. Elevated PbBs have been found in 1–12% of the samples analyzed from the screening probes. The highest incidences were found in Lenoir and New Hanover counties, which were selected for one of our studies.

Local Screening Programs

Pb screening in most areas of North Carolina is carried out as an optional part of the EPSDT Program. Lenoir, Cabarrus, New Hanover,

SCREENING PROCEDURE

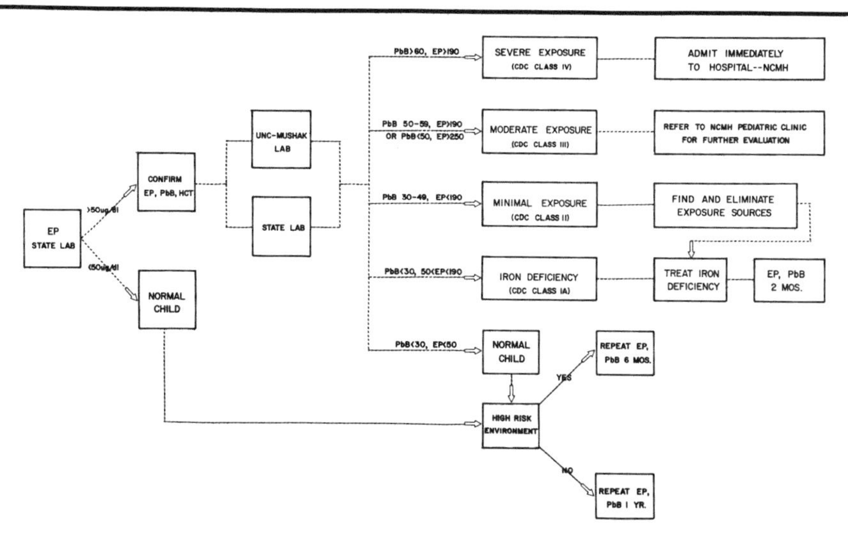

FIGURE 1. Screening procedures for the Lead Screening Program.

and Wake Counties, however, have organized aggressive screening, intervention, and abatement programs in response to recent outbreaks of Pb poisoning in these areas. Subjects for our early studies were referred primarily by the Wake County Health Department and we continued to study these children. We also studied children from more remote parts of the state by means of a mobile laboratory in Lenoir and New Hanover counties.

Pb-Industry Target Populations

A variety of major Pb industries are located in North Carolina. Children whose parents work in these industries constitute a discrete population with increased risk of lead poisoning. Permission was obtained to continue the study of children from families employed by one of these Pb industries. About half of the subjects who participated in our initial study were obtained from this source. These children constituted a large part of the five-year follow-up study. It should be noted that the study population consisted of a self-selected sample from the lower income segment of the general population; we felt that concentration on the lower income group was appropriate in this project because lead poisoning is most prevalent in this target group (see U.S. EPA, 1977, 1986).

Experimental Design and Statistical Methodology

These were not experimental studies, but rather used a cross-sectional observational epidemiologic design. No manipulation of independent variables was made. In other words, we assumed for purposes of hypothesis testing a random sample representative of children likely to be considered for screening for lead exposure in the EPSDT population.

The principal approach to analysis involved multiple regression modelling with age and PbB as predictors for Central Nervous System (CNS) outcomes. When considering IQ as the outcome, the regression models controlled for age, SES, Home Environment Score, and maternal IQ. The general strategy for determining the best model paralleled the approach of Kleinbaum, Kupper, and Morgenstern (1982).

Lead Analysis Procedures

An essential part of toxicology research is the assessment of the amount of a toxic substance present in a given system. In this research, blood lead level was the key predictor variable under study. Measurements of blood lead and lead in house paint and house dust were the responsibility of the Heavy Metals Analysis Laboratory, Department of Pathology, University of North Carolina at Chapel Hill (UNC-Chapel Hill). The laboratory had a variety of trace analytical equipment, including atomic absorpting spectrometers (AAS) that permit both flame and flameless atomic absorption analysis.

Lead in Blood

The Delves Cup micro procedure (Delves, 1970) with the modification by Ediger and Coleman (1972) was employed for whole blood (and plasma) lead determinations. The Delves Cup procedure was selected on the basis of speed, minimal sample manipulation, and concomitant low contamination risk and a good "track record" in our hands and in other laboratories. Speed was a critical factor because of the large volume blood analysis requirements and relative instability of blood. Direct insertion of blood samples into Delves Cups followed by drying, preignition, and atomization of the contained lead is rapid and relatively free from contamination problems. A number of interlaboratory method comparison studies have shown the Delves Cup micro procedure to be as good as or better than other atomic absorption or nonatomic absorption techniques. Furthermore, this procedure is used by many laboratories in the CDC proficiency screening program.

Special precautions were taken to minimize sample contamination prior to analysis. All glassware that came in contact with samples was washed and chemically debrided of metal contaminants by low-metal acid washing followed by repeated deionized water rinsing. Reagents, solvents for reagents, and other assay materials were selected for very small or undectectable metal contaminant content. With human subjects, blood was collected into B-D low-lead vacutainer tubes via puncture.

Quality control was maintained by both internal and external means. Frequent preparation and testing of aqueous and matrix-matched standards on a daily or weekly basis was employed to assess changes in day-to-day precision and accuracy. External monitoring of laboratory performance was achieved by participation of our laboratory in the CDC's proficiency testing for blood lead determination. Further methodology evaluation was done using certified blood samples of known metal content and provided either by a commercial source (Kaulson Laboratories) or by the New York State Health Department. In the CDC program, three month bovine samples were airmailed to our laboratory and analyzed and the results forwarded to CDC. Our results were then compared both with overall participant performance and with the mean values for the reference laboratories. Our overall performance has been quite good over the range of blood lead levels encountered in the proficiency survey.

Instrument and Test Battery Development

This project had several unique features: the development of a mobile neurotoxicity testing laboratory that permitted the assessment of children in remote cachement areas with sophisticated behavioral and electrophysiological measures; a cooperative arrangement with federal, state, county, and local health agencies and industry that permitted the coordinated screening and assessment of at risk children across the state; and an opportunity to obtain valuable longitudinal data on the long-term effects of early Pb exposure on neurobehavioral and cognitive development. This project was based on a productive collaboration among the EPA, the University of North Carolina School of Medicine, the North Carolina Division of Health Services, and private industry. The addition of a sophisticated mobile laboratory for the assessment of exposure significantly enhanced the research capabilities of the team.

Behavioral and medical evaluations were carried out by professional staff from the Division for Disorders of Development and Learning (DDDL). DDDL is a clinical training facility that is part of the Child

Development Research Institute and Biological Sciences Research Center (BSRC) at the University of North Carolina.

Daily Test Protocal and Home Visit

Collection of electrophysiological data was done at DDDL or in the field mobile laboratory. Demographic, psychometric, and medical data were obtained in an auxiliary trailer or in space provided by local health agencies.

Families were seen for a testing protocol that took approximately four hours to complete. Informed consent was obtained from the parent(s), who also were asked to sign a volunteer's statement. At the time of testing, the examiner was blind as to the child's lead exposure. A maximum of four children per day could be evaluated in the mobile laboratory.

After evaluation day a home visit was made for several reasons. If behavior problems were assumed to be related to lead exposure, control assessments of the home environment would have to be made to estimate its contribution to the child's hyperactivity or any other problem behavior. The Caldwell HOME Inventory is a standardized rating scale used for this purpose. The home was evaluated as a vehicle for continued lead exposure; the lead, if discovered, had to be removed by cleaning supervised by the county health department. Dust samples from the living room carpet, bedroom, and inside the front door were obtained by suction on preweighed glass filters and analyzed for lead by x-ray fluorescence using a portable unit. Home water supply was also analyzed for lead by AAS. These analyses have led to clean up of several homes and a resultant reduction of PbB levels of the lead-exposed children (Milar & Mushak, 1982). Once all the clinical data were gathered and evaluated, the children were reviewed at a staffing conference and any problems discovered during evaluation, whether they were lead related or not, were referred to the appropriate local community resources for follow-up. Children with PbB > 50 μg/dl and FEP > 190 μg/dl were referred to a hospital for further evaluation and treatment of elevated lead levels.

Medical, Psychometric, and Behavioral Measures

Table 3 summarizes the blood lead chemistry and medical, electrophysiological, psychometric, behavioral, and demographic measures that were collected from children and parents who participated in this project. These measures were chosen to provide convergent information from several different perspectives in order to elaborate more clearly the subtle and complex effects of asymptomatic lead exposure on CNS development.

TABLE 3

Summary of Evaluations

I. *Exposure Evaluation*
   A. Fantus Lead Poisoning Questionnaire
   B. Blood lead (PbB): flameless atomic absorption spectrometry
   C. Free erythrocyte protoporphyrin (FEP)

II. *Medical Evaluation*
   A. Medical history
   B. Pediatric neurological examination
   C. Growth: height, weight, head circumference
   D. Lab tests: BDS, WBC, RBC, Hgb, HCT, MCV, MCH, MCHC

III. *Electrophysiological Evaluation*
   A. Slow Cortical Potentials during Sensory Conditioning
   B. Brainstem Auditory Evoked Potentials
   C. Pattern-Reversal Visual Evoked Potentials

IV. *Psychometric-Behavioral Evaluation*
   A. Stanford-Binet Intelligence Test—Revised
   B. Bayley Scales of Infant Development (<30 mos. of age)

V. *Demographic Covariate Evaluation*
   A. Maternal IQ: Ammons Quick Test or Peabody Picture Vocabulary Test Revised
   B. Socioeconomic status: Hollingshead Two-Factor Index
   C. Quality of caregiving environment: Caldwell's Home Observation for Measurement of the Environment
   D. Chronological age
   E. Sex

Several tests were selected on the basis of guidelines that were later adopted at an International Symposium on Neurobehavioal Methodology in Pediatric Lead Research held in Cincinnati in September, 1981. These guidelines included: (a) use of standardized, age-normed tests with documented validity and reliability when available; (b) use of experimental measures to evaluate areas of function for which standardized measures are not available; and (c) use of instruments with cross-cultural comparison data.

An extensive medical history was taken on each child to rule out a variety of problems related to mental retardation but not attributable to lead, and to evaluate lead exposure history. The instrument we used was the *Lead Poisoning Study Questionnaire* developed at the Fantus Lead Screening Clinic at Cook County Hospital in Chicago. This 28-page questionnaire examines pertinent demographic history, prenatal history, child developmental milestones, past medical history, lead poisoning symptomatology, dietary history, family history, immunizations, illnesses, vital signs, and chelation therapy and side effects.

STUDY I: COMPARISON OF CHILDREN OCCUPATIONALLY AND NONOCCUPATIONALLY EXPOSED TO LEAD

From 1975 to 1980, we conducted an interdisciplinary lead screening program as part of a program project grant from the National Institute of Environmental Health Sciences (ES-01104). Our strategy was to screen a population not only with traditional psychometric measures, but also for subclinical dose related effects of lead using direct longitudinal observations of children's behavior, for example, home observations, parent/child interactions, activity level, and slow wave brain potentials that might be developmentally related to subclinical lead levels and the children's behavior. Such a strategy, with appropriate design, might allow a search for behavioral threshold effects of lead while avoiding the criticisms of previous studies.

A North Carolina Memorial Hospital case report of lead poisoning in a family from Raleigh uncovered a highly stable and cooperative population associated with a battery factory in Wake County, where the relatives were employed. The children were exposed to lead dust brought home and deposited in the house dust and in the carpets, which placed toddlers at the crawling stage at risk (Dolcourt, 1977; Dolcourt, Hamrick, O'Tuama, Wooten, & Baker, 1978). From 1977 to 1979, we evaluated over 115 children, 42 of whom were children of employees in that plant and 104 of whom met criteria for study. We continue to follow them longitudinally.

Methods

Subjects

One hundred and four children in Wake County aged 10 months to 6 1/2 years at the time of initial testings who met inclusion criteria served as subjects. They were mostly black (94%) from lower social classes—that is, x=4.5 on the Hollingshead Two-Factor Index (Hollingshead, 1957). Children previously evidencing CNS disease or insult or having undergone chelation therapy for lead poisoning and children with prediagnosed language delay or mental retardation were excluded from data analysis. Approximately half of the children were less than 30 months of age and half were over 30 months of age. Half of the subjects were EPSDT children and half were children of battery factory workers referred from a local county health department to the lead screening program at North Carolina Memorial Hospital as part of a statewide screening program.

Procedures

Subjects were evaluated at DDDL in the protocol described above in *General Methodolgy,* except that the only electrophysiological measures they received were Slow Cortical Potentials during Sensory Conditioning (see Otto et al., 1981, for a report of results).

Results and Discussion

A preliminary forward stepwise regression analysis of the relationship of lead to IQ and 18 of the covariates showed no effect of occupational exposure among the present cohort of children (Hawk & Schroeder, 1983). Therefore, further analysis of occupational exposure was dropped and the number of confounding variables was reduced to HOME, SES, maternal IQ, age, sex, test (Bayley versus Stanford-Binet), presence of the father in the home, and number of siblings, in order to avoid overcontrol and Type II errors. The main statistical model used a multivariate regression analysis in which a set of all the interaction terms was tested first. If the set were nonsignificant, all interactions were dropped from the model. The second step was to test the main effects of the confounding variables. Finally, the test for the main effects of lead was performed. Any significant result was then further reduced in a stepwise manner for individual or linear combinations of variables for inclusion in the final model (Kleinbaum et al., 1982).

The main result was that there was a significant linear relationship between blood lead level (range 6–59 μg/dl) and IQ ($F = 7.689$; df 1, 96, $p < .01$) (Figure 2). None of the interaction terms nor any of the quadratic or cubic effects was significant. Of the confounding variables only SES was significant ($F = 20.159$; df 1, 96, $p < .001$) and remained in the model. Nevertheless, the main effect of lead on IQ remained significant.

The failure of HOME, maternal IQ, and age to reach significance as they had in other studies was likely the result of multicollinearity with SES. Table 4 shows that the intercorrelation of these variables was high. It seems that whichever of these variables enters the regression equation first is likely to render the effects of the others less significant. While SES and HOME shared a great deal of variance, one would ordinarily expect a direct measure of caregiving environment like the HOME to be a more accurate measure than an indirect one based on parental occupation and education like SES. Order of entry of multicollinear covariates into the regression equation was important in determining which were significant and which were not. We will return to the matter of separating the effects of social factors on the relationship between lead and IQ in the *Study III: Replication Study*.

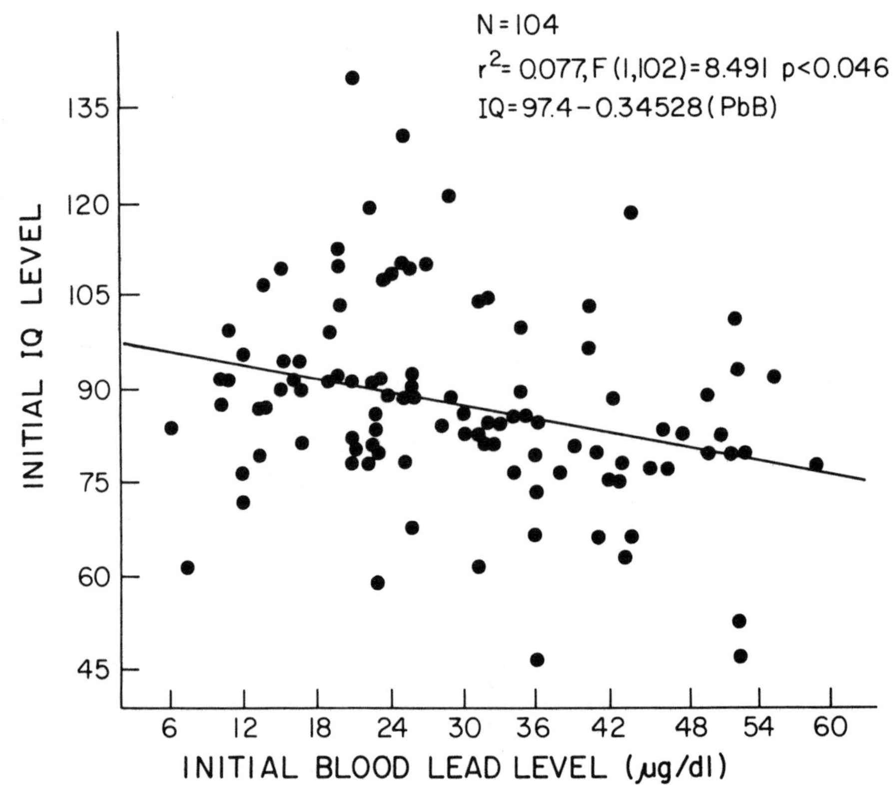

FIGURE 2. Initial IQ as a function of initial blood lead levels of children screened from 1977–1979.

TABLE 4

Correlation Matrix of Blood Lead Level and Child IQ (1977) and Comcomitant Variables

VARIABLES	PbB	IQ	HOME	MatIQ	CA	SEX	SES	FaPr
Blood lead level (PbB)								
Child IQ	−.276							
Caldwell HOME	−.269	.451						
Maternal IQ (MatIQ)	−.193	.379	.522					
Chronological age (CA)	−.068	.254	.089	.029				
Sex	−.072	.130	.123	−.028	.062			
Socioeconomic status (SES)	.183	−.449	−.624	−.475	−.143	−.064		
Father present (FaPr)	−.010	.165	.433	.178	.161	.054	−.495	
Number of siblings (Sibs)	.314	−.284	−.202	−.177	.116	−.003	.161	−.064

STUDY II: FIVE-YEAR FOLLOW-UP STUDY

The basic objective of this study (Schroeder, Hawk, Otto, Mushak, & Hicks, 1985) was to determine whether asymptomatic lead exposure in early childhood resulted in residual altered CNS function in children when they reached school age. There might be latent or cumulative effects, even though their blood lead levels would be lower because they had grown out of the toddler stage.

Methods

Subjects

Eighty of the 104 children from Study I were located through county health department and school records five years later in 1983. Of the 80, 50 agreed to reevaluation.

Procedures

Children were seen at the Wake County Health Department in the mobile laboratory using the same protocol as in Study I, described under *General Methodology*, except that the home visit was not repeated. Most of their blood lead levels had come down (Figure 3).

Results and Discussion

The same logistic backward multiple regression analysis was used as in the initial study except that initial blood lead level was used as the independent variable, current blood lead level was added to the list of covariates, and test and age were dropped as covariates because all of the children received the Stanford-Binet IQ test this time. The two lead scores were highly correlated ($r = 0.74$); the correlation of initial lead to follow-up IQ was also significant ($r = 0.34$, $p < .05$).

The main result in this study was that in the regression analysis lead no longer had a significant effect after the confounding variables were added to the model ($F < 1$). Apparently, the decline in lead levels, while not appreciably disturbing the relation of social factors to lead and IQ, did negate lead's relation to IQ when confounding factors were controlled. This was not caused by self-selection bias at follow-up because the demographic characteristics of the families who participated were very similar to those who did not.

In conclusion, in the present cohort of mainly low SES black families, the covariance matrix among social factors and the relationship of lead to

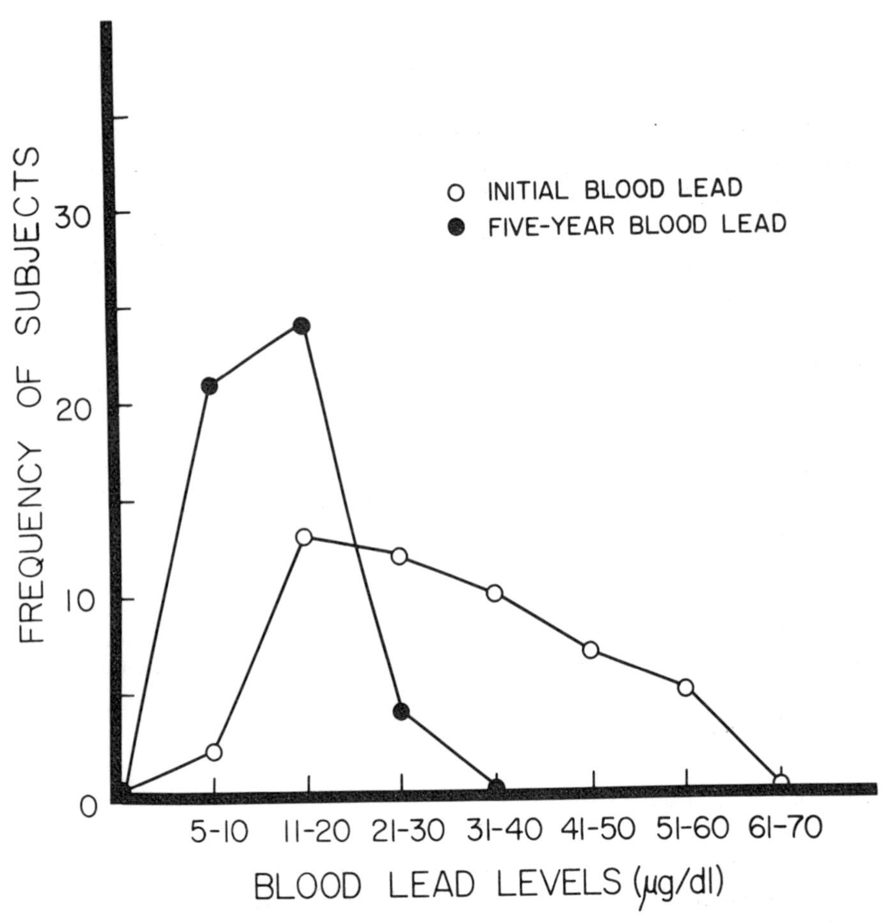

FIGURE 3. Frequency distribution of blood lead levels of children seen from 1977–1978 and in follow-up five years later.

IQ seemed to be fairly stable over a five-year period. SES seemed to capture much of the variance related to the other covariates because of multicollinearity with HOME, maternal IQ, and age.

STUDY III: REPLICATION STUDY

The primary objectives of this study were to replicate the previous studies in a more homogenous group (all-black low SES children aged 3–7 years) and to find the best regression model based on both accuracy and precision that described the relationship of lead and IQ (Hawk et al., 1985). Regression analyses typically eliminate or incorporate control variables on the basis of *precision*, that is, whether significant additional variation in one's outcome variable is explained by adding one or more control variables to the model comprised of outcome and predictor variables. Alternatively, an unforced backward regression would eliminate all variables that do not account for a significant amount of variance with the outcome variable. Precision is concerned with random error, that is, the size of the confidence interval around the estimated parameter, that can occur when estimating effects. *Confounding*, on the other hand, is concerned with systematic error that can occur when estimating effects. Confounding is said to exist (Kleinbaum et al., 1982) if a meaningfully different interpretation of the relationship of interest will result, depending on whether an extraneous variable is ignored or included in one's data analysis.

Confounding, then, is concerned with the issue of validity, that is, whether one has the right answer. Kleinbaum et al. (1982) suggested an analogy to target shooting: validity (confounding) is concerned with whether or not one is aiming at the correct bull's eye, while precision is concerned with individual variation from shot to shot, given the actual bull's eye involved. According to Kleinbaum et al. (1982), while both precision and confounding must be considered and incorporated during the modeling process, for etiologic questions (such as the questions addressed in this study) confounding, or validity, usually takes final precedence over precision in the determination of the final model. These issues were addressed in the replication.

Methods

Subjects

Eighty black children aged 3–7 were recruited from high risk neighborhoods in Lenoir and New Hanover counties in cooperation with county health agencies and the Environmental Epidemiology Branch (EEB) of the North Carolina Division of Health Services. Most of the members of the New Hanover sample were enrolled in the Headstart Program. A list of criteria that defined the eligibility of individual children for inclusion in the study was provided to referring health agencies. Eligibility criteria are specified below.

1. Age	3–7 years
2. Race	Black
3. Health status/history	Subjects could not have any current acute or chronic illness or be under medication of any sort. Perinatal his-

	tory should be free of complications. Subjects should not have any history of neurobiological insults.
4. Lead exposure history	Child should be asymptomatic and never have received chelation therapy or been treated for lead poisoning. A range of PbB levels from 5–60 μg/dl was desired.
5. Socioeconomic status	Only low income families defined as Class IV or V (Hollingshead Scale) were included. EPSDT families were included in this group.
6. IQ	In order to exclude any children who were clearly mentally retarded, a minimum subject IQ of 60 was required.

Procedures

The same procedures as outlined in the General Methodology section were performed. Based on the results of our previous studies, covariates in the present study were restricted to HOME, SES, maternal IQ, age, and gender.

Results and Discussion

Of the 80 children screened, 75 met the inclusion criteria and were used for analysis. Their demographic characteristics are given in Table 5. The mean socioeconomic status of this group was lower than other groups that we have studied. Also, the low maternal intelligence scores reflect the

TABLE 5

Demographic Characteristics of Children in the Replication Study

DEMOGRAPHIC CHARACTERISTICS	MEAN SCORE	SD	RANGE
Mean blood lead level (μg/dl)	21.80	9.76	6.00–39.00
High blood lead level (μg/dl)	26.71	14.11	6.20–56.00
Most recent blood lead level (μg/dl)	20.65	9.73	6.20–47.40
Most recent FEP (μg/dl)	32.74	14.03	8.0 –193.0
Home caregiver practices (Bradley & Caldwell, 1976a, 1979b)	59.84	15.08	20–87
Maternal IQ (Dunn & Dunn, 1981)	63.41	11.29	40–94
Chronological age (mos.)	58.40	11.74	39–94
Socioeconomic class (Hollingshead Two-Factor Index)	4.91	0.20	4–5

new revised norms for the Peabody Picture Vocabulary Test, Revised (PPVT-R) (Dunn & Dunn, 1981), which are less comparable to the more common adult intelligence tests such as the Wechsler Adult Intelligence Scale (WAIS), but which are perhaps more valid than the Ammons Quick Test.

STATISTICAL ANALYSIS STRATEGY FOR ASSESSING INTERACTION AND CONFOUNDING OF SOCIAL FACTORS

The main objective of the statistical analysis strategy was to find the model that best described the relationship between lead and IQ. The principal approach to analysis involved multiple regression modeling with blood lead level as a predictor variable, child IQ as the outcome variable, and age, SES, HOME score, gender, and maternal IQ as control variables. The control variables were restricted to those five that had proven significant in our earlier studies in order to reduce Type II errors caused by overcontrol. Type I errors were controlled by focusing on one confirmatory hypothesis—that blood lead levels would be significantly related to child IQ—while controlling for SES, maternal IQ, HOME (caregiving environment), gender, and age. Exploratory analyses were performed to find the most accurate and precise model that described the relationship between lead and IQ and their covariates.

Methods

The general strategy for determining the best regression model was the same hierarchical logistic modeling strategy of Kleinbaum et al. (1982) as was used before. This strategy incorporated the assessment of confounding, interaction, and precision into the selection of variables for the final model. A backward stepwise multiple regression approach was used in which interactions (PbB × age, PbB × SES, PbB × MIQ, PbB × HOME) were tested first, followed by the set of possible confounding covariate effects, followed by examination of main effects of lead and IQ. This approach involved testing for a set of variables (e.g., all the interaction terms) in an overall test (chunk test) rather than testing for individual variables at each step, to enhance the simplicity and interpretability of the final model. Tests that attained significance or near significance were then followed by stepdown (backward stepwise regression) tests to identify specific variables that should be retained in the final model to increase its precision. If the overall test results were not significant, these terms were dropped from the final model. However, simply using stepwise regression to obtain a best regression model can lead to misleading interpretation of data because the issue of confounding is not automatically addressed by such analyses (Kleinbaum et al., 1982).

Exploratory analyses were then performed to find the most accurate *and* precise model. A variable (e.g., age, SES, etc.) determined to be a nonconfounder might still be retained in the model to increase *precision;* that is, the variable might significantly contribute to the total variability in IQ over and above what is contributed by the other variables remaining in the model. Similarly, even though confounding may be present within a set of variables, it may be that some smaller subset is all that is required for control, while providing increased precision in estimating the association of interest.

Procedures

Finding the model that best described the data in terms of both precision and confounding was accomplished in the following way. A *gold standard,* that is, a baseline or standard adjusted estimate of association, was compared with adjusted estimates of association that accounted for other combinations of the extraneous variables. The gold standard was the model obtained in the backward regression analysis that controlled for all interactions but kept all the control variables in the model. A subset of these variables that gave nearly the same adjusted estimates of the regression coefficient ($\hat{\beta}$) for PbB was then a candidate for selection.

The first model to be compared to this gold standard was obtained in the backward regression that eliminated control variables in terms of precision (finding the factors that explained the most variability in the dependent variable). This answered the question of whether the most precise model was also the most valid model. If the two models were not the same (i.e., the most precise model was *not* the most valid model), other models were chosen based on logic, predictions from past literature, and examination of the steps of the original backward elimination. The $\hat{\beta}$ coefficients obtained from these various general linear models were compared to the gold standard and those most similar were then used to calculate confidence intervals for each model. The formula used for this calculation was as follows: $\hat{\beta}$ + (^{T}64, .975) (S$\hat{\beta}$). The model with the smallest confidence interval is the model with the greatest precision, that is, the most accurate and precise model.

Results and Discussion

IQ Results

Results of the confirmatory univariate analysis of the relation of current blood lead level to IQ are shown in the summary table (Table 6) below. Since the chunk test of interactions and control variables were nonsignificant, each set was dropped from the model. Exploratory tests using maximal (historically highest level obtained from Public Health Department records) and mean PbB levels were also done to further clarify the effect. Table 6 shows that there was a very strong negative linear relationship between blood lead levels and IQ, irrespective of which PbB index was used. Results of tests for quadratic and cubic components were not significant. Figure 4 shows a smooth linear relationship between the highest (47.4 μg/dl) and the lowest (6.3 μg/dl) blood lead levels.

Results of the Exploratory Analyses

Although the multiple regression analysis for the interaction terms using the overall chunk test was not significant, the one for control variables approached significance, suggesting that a more accurate and precise model could be found. Furthermore, inspection of Table 7 shows that, while the regression model with lead and IQ alone (including no covariates) was the most precise, that is, had the smallest confidence interval, the coefficient for lead differed considerably from that of the gold standard, that is, the model that included lead, IQ, SES, HOME, maternal IQ, age, and gender. Therefore, stepdown backward regression analyses were performed in which each variable was considered individually. No interaction variables were found to be significant, even when considered individually in the backward stepwise regression. When backward regression continued using all single independent variables (e.g., PbB and control variables) with no forcing, SES was the first variable to be eliminated, followed by age, gender, and then HOME, while maternal IQ

TABLE 6

Summary Table of the Confirmatory Analysis of the Relation of Blood Lead & IQ Univariate F, p

		STANFORD-BINET IQ TEST	
EFFECT	USING CURRENT PbB	USING MEAN PbB	USING HIGHEST PbB
Interactions	0.55, 0.74	1.01, 0.42	1.34, 0.26
Control	1.82, 012	1.86, 0.11	1.76, 0.13
Lead PbB	12.31, 0.0008	10.08, 0.002	10.55, 0.0018
R	0.144	0.121	0.126

remained in the model with lead. Lead and maternal IQ were found to be significant variables in relationship to child IQ. That is, the model that included only those variables sharing a significant amount of variance with the dependent variable was the model comprised of lead and maternal IQ.

However, comparison of the coefficient for lead in this model (IQ, lead, and maternal IQ) with the gold standard (from the stepwise regression that eliminated all interactions but kept all single variables) indicated that there was a discrepancy between their values that seemed to be substantial (Table 7). Therefore, other models employing different combinations of terms were examined (IQ, PbB, SES, maternal IQ, HOME; IQ, PbB, age, maternal IQ, HOME, gender; IQ, PbB, maternal IQ, HOME; IQ, PbB, maternal IQ, HOME, gender). Similarity of their coefficients for lead to that of the gold standard were assessed and sizes of the confidence intervals were calculated for each. The model with the smallest difference in $\hat{\beta}$ coefficient for lead from that of the gold standard that still maintained a small confidence interval was IQ, PbB, maternal IQ, HOME, and gender. That is, the model that best controlled for confounding with the greatest precision (i.e., the most accurate and

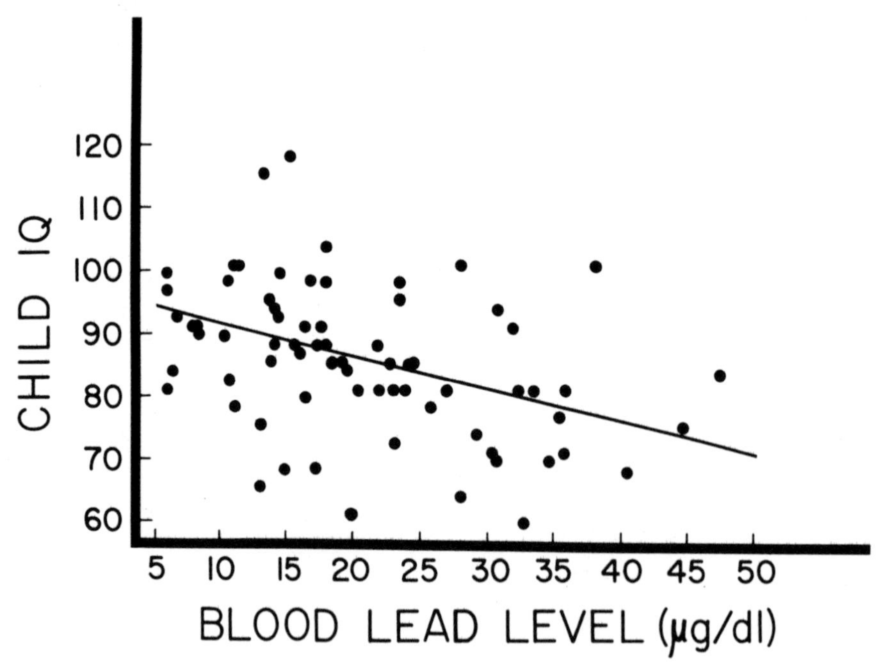

FIGURE 4. Child IQ as a function of blood lead levels of children screened in the replication study.

precise model) contained lead, maternal IQ, HOME, and gender. Nevertheless two other models (IQ, PbB, age, gender, HOME, and maternal IQ; IQ, PbB, gender, HOME, and maternal IQ) gave acceptable accuracy and precision. All the models in Table 7 were significant beyond the $p<.01$ level.

The exploratory analyses demonstrated two important points: the most precise regression model may not always be the most accurate one in the assessment of confounding social factors on the lead-IQ relation; and if both precision and accuracy are considered, then HOME environment was more precise and accurate than SES in the population studied. SES is a rather crude measure that may not accurately reflect the heterogeneity of caregiving practices among lower SES families (Dietrich et al., 1985; Elardo, Bradley, & Caldwell, 1975; Ramey, Farran, & Campbell, 1979; White & Watts, 1973). Indeed the relation of HOME score to SES may be different for different social classes. Recently, Bellinger, Needleman, Leviton, Waternaux, Rabinowitz, and Nichols (1984) found that HOME scores were positively related to umbilical cord blood lead levels in upper middle and upper class inner city Boston families, just the opposite of what has been found with lower SES families. Therefore, SES and HOME are not interchangeable measures. Considerably more study of their interrelationships is needed. The present study suggests that assessments

TABLE 7

Accuracy and Precision of Different Models of Regression of Blood Lead Levels on IQ Including Different Combinations of Variables as Candidates for Control Variables

CANDIDATE SUBSET	β COEFFICIENT[a]	95% CONFIDENCE INTERVAL $[\hat{\beta} \pm (t64,975)(S\,\hat{\beta})]$		
1. Age,SES,Gender,HOME,MIQ,PbB,IQ[e]	−0.254	0.049[b]	−0.558[c]	0.607[d]
2. Age, Gender,HOME,MIQ,PbB,IQ	−0.248	0.051	−0.548	0.598
3. SES, HOME,MIQ,PbB,IQ	−0.282	0.021	−0.585	0.606
4. Gender,HOME,MIQ,PbB,IQ[f]	−0.255	0.043	−0.554	0.597
5. HOME,MIQ,PbB,IQ	−0.273	0.026	−0.572	0.598
6. MIQ,PbB,IQ	−0.396	−0.102	−0.637	0.535
7. PbB,IQ	−0.456	−0.196	−0.715	0.520

[a]This is the β coefficient for lead
[b]Lower bound of the confidence interval
[c]Upper bound of the confidence interval
[d]Absolute difference between the lower and upper bounds of the confidence interval
[e]The baseline model or *gold standard* with all control variables included
[f]The match to the gold standard with least confounding (β coefficient for lead that is closest to that in the *gold standard*) while maintaining good precision (small confidence interval)

of their precision *and* accuracy are important criteria to consider in choosing the best regression model for lead and IQ.

GENERAL DISCUSSION

Lead Exposure and IQ in Children

Considerable controversy exists concerning the effects of low to moderate Pb exposure on cognitive function, as indexed by standard IQ tests, in children (U.S. EPA, 1986). Results of the replication study provide very strong evidence ($p < .001$) in young children of a continuous linear decrease in IQ (Stanford-Binet Full Scale) with increasing blood lead level across a wide range (5–47 μg/dl). This confirmatory finding is particularly compelling because the potentially confounding factor of socioeconomic status was effectively controlled by selecting a very homogeneous group of children (mostly SES Class V).

Results of the five-year follow-up study provided further clarification of the long-term effect of Pb exposure on IQ. Initial assessment of these children aged 1–6 in 1977–1978 showed the same inverse linear relationship of PbB and IQ as found in the replication study. In addition, a dissociation of maternal and child IQ (Perino & Ernhart, 1974) was found ($r = 0.058$) in children below 30 months of age with elevated PbB levels (≥ 30 μg/dl). Five years later the PbB levels of all children retested had dropped to ≤ 30 μg/dl. After controlling for possible confounding variables (SES and HOME caregiver scores), no significant Pb effect on IQ was apparent and the previously observed dissociation of maternal and child IQ was no longer present ($r = 0.451$). These observations suggest that IQ decrements associated with undue Pb absorption in the low to moderate range may be reversible if appropriate abatement procedures are taken to reduce body Pb burdens in young children. However, these children must be followed into adulthood to seriously test this hypothesis.

Assessing the Effects of the Caregiving Environment and Other Social Factors

In all of the present studies, socioeconomic status, maternal IQ, and HOME scores were highly interrelated. The combination of these three covariates seems to be at the source of multiple pathways that affect the relationship between lead exposure and IQ. It seems that a variety of social factors must be considered for a given population and that a considerable amount of additional research will be needed before the pieces can all be fitted into the mosaic that will yield a coherent picture of these interrelationships. Below we consider some of the main interrelationships of the social covariates of lead exposure in children.

HOME Scores

In the current research HOME scores were consistently related to maternal IQ, SES, and presence of the father in the home (see Table 4). This last variable was also highly related to SES. Father absence was probably more of a socioeconomic variable in that it was related to the mother's receiving public assistance. A related effect was that single mothers and their children often lived with relatives as part of an extended family resource network. Families who lacked these other breadwinners tended to be more indigent and more socially isolated.

The relation of HOME scores to blood lead level also seems to vary with age. Milar et al. (1980) found a significant relationship of HOME scores to blood lead levels and Bayley MDI scores in the 11–30 month age range, but not in the 31–72 month range. Dietrich et al. (1985) found, in a comparable inner city population in Cincinnati, a significant relationship of neonatal umbilical cord blood lead levels and HOME scores, which tended to increase from 1 to 15 months of age. However, this is just the opposite of what Bellinger et al. (1984) found in an upper middle and upper class white population in a renovated inner city Boston area. So it seems that there may be a complex age × SES × race interaction with HOME scores that may be related to exposure to lead and its relationship to IQ.

Socioeconomic Status

Does SES protect or compensate for developmental risk caused by pre- and perinatal neurotoxic insults like lead exposure? In the present experiments, and certainly in most of the experiments discussed in Table 1, SES tended to account for a great deal of the variance found in the relationship between lead and IQ. However, as discussed above, this seems to depend greatly on the age, sex, and race of the population studied. SES is a passive, rather crude measure of caregiving environment. Studies by Sameroff and Chandler (1975) indicate that SES can indeed buffer physiological insults in the pre- and perinatal period. However, this may not always be the case, given the nature of some neurotoxic risks. For example, Bellinger et al. (1984) found a positive relationship between HOME score and umbilical cord lead in an upper middle and upper class white population living in a newly renovated inner city Boston area. Thus, in this case high SES placed children at a higher risk for lead exposure (from the dust from the lead paint on old buildings that had been torn down or sandblasted). Further, caregiving practices per se may be overshadowed in such a setting by the risks associated with housing environments chosen as a result of having a high socioeconomic status. On the other hand, White (1982), in a meta-analysis of 200 studies relating SES to academic achievement, found that a much higher correlation between home atmosphere and academic achievement than in any other combination of SES indicators. The more important variables were childrearing practices and stimulation of learning at home and at school, and not parents' occupation, income, or education. Children living in socially disadvantaged settings may have fewer opportunities for such experiences, but this does not automatically confer adverse risk upon them. Rather, the risk seems to lie in the combination of HOME, SES, and maternal IQ.

Maternal IQ

In the present studies maternal IQ was highly related to HOME scores, SES, and child IQ in Experiments I, II, and III and with blood lead level in experiment III ($r = 0.314$, $p < .007$). There was a great deal of heterogeneity among the mothers of the children in the current studies, both in intellectual level and in childrearing practices. Many of the mothers were very conscientious, but others engaged in harsh disciplinary practices and provided only a minimum of stimulation for their children in the home. HOME scores ranged from 20–87 in Study III, for instance (see Table 5). In particular, the most indigent mothers displayed depression, showing little positive affect toward their children. Dietrich et al. (1985) also reported a lack of emotional responsivity of caregivers, which was related to lack of child supervision and to lead exposure.

Maternal IQ may also be related to neglect of children's nutritional needs. In the present studies nutrition was controlled by excluding from study those subjects with nutritional deficiencies, such as iron deficiencies. But in everyday life there are many ways in which borderline nutritional deficiencies may affect lead exposure (Milar & Schroeder, 1983): (a) by serving as a nutritional basis for pica (Snowdon, 1977); (b) by altering susceptibility to lead intoxication because of deficiencies in iron, copper, chromium, zinc, calcium, and Vitamin D, all of which compete with lead for protein binding sites (Mahaffey & Michaelson, 1980); (c) because of persistence of mouthing and pica of people with mental retardation or autism into adulthood (Danford & Huber, 1982).

Multiple Paths and Expressions of Neurotoxic Effects of Lead

There are many paths by which social factors can affect the relationship between lead and IQ. Certainly IQ is by far the most well studied neurotoxic effect of lead exposure in children. However, there are other effects of lead exposure, such as fine motor, perceptual-motor, reaction time, sensory-neural, and evoked and slow wave potential electrophysiological effects, which have also been demonstrated and for which the effects of social factors have hardly been studied. There are also many other stressful biological effects of lead, for example, hematological, nephrological, cardiovascular, endocrine, and gastroenterological effects, whose interaction with neurotoxic effects have not been addressed at all. Such a complex view of neurotoxicity renders it difficult to study (Weiss, 1980). Indeed Bornschein (1985) has criticized traditional *main effects* models as inadequate for reflecting the complexity of human neurotoxicity. In his view, a dynamic interactional longitudinal model as illustrated in the use of structural equations is preferable. However, such models will also have to cope with such sources of error as sampling, attrition, history, maturation, different test instruments for different age groups, statistical regression, heterogeneity of covariates over time, etc. (Baltes & Nesselroade, 1979). For instance, SES might be fairly stable over time in a low SES group caught in the poverty cycle, but quite different in an upwardly mobile middle class group. Such a change might easily affect the relationship of lead exposure to IQ over time. Nevertheless, longitudinal studies will likely provide more conclusive answers to the many questions concerning the neurotoxic effects of lead on retardation of cognitive and adaptive development.

REFERENCES

Alexander, F.W., Delves, H.T., & Clayton, B.E. (1972). The uptake and excretion by children of lead and other contaminants. In D. Barth et al. (Eds.), *Environmental health aspects of lead: Proceedings of an international symposium* (pp. 319–330). Amsterdam: Commission of the European Communities.

Baltes, P.B., & Nesselroade, J.R. (1979). History and rationale of longitudinal research. In J.R. Nesselroade & P.B. Baltes (Eds.), *Longitudinal research in the study of behavior and development* (pp. 1–39). New York: Academic Press.

Bayley, N. (1970). Development of mental abilities. In L. Carmichael (Ed.), *Manual of child psychology* (3rd ed.). New York: Wiley.

Bellinger, D.C., Needleman, H.L., Leviton, A., Waternaux, C., Rabinowitz, M.B., & Nichols, M.L. (1984). Early sensory-motor development and prenatal exposure to lead. *Neurobehavioral Toxicology and Teratology, 6,* 387–402.

Bornschein, R.L. (1985). Influence of social factors on lead exposure and child development. Paper submitted for publication.

Bradley, R., & Caldwell, B. (1976a). Early home environment and changes in mental test performance in children from 6 to 36 months. *Developmental Psychology, 12,* 93–97.

Bradley, R. & Caldwell, B. (1976b). The relation of infants' home environments to mental test performance at fifty-four months: A follow-up study. *Child Development, 47,* 1172–1174.

Bradley, R., & Caldwell, B. (1979a). Early home environment and changes in mental test performance in children from 6–36 months. *Developmental Psychology, 12,* 93–97.

Bradley, R., & Caldwell, B. (1979b). Home Observation for Measurement of the

Environment: A revision of the preschool scale. *American Journal of Mental Deficiency, 84,* 235–244.
Caldwell, B., & Bradley, R. (1979). *Home observation for measurement of the environment: Administration manual.* University of Arkansas at Little Rock.
Caldwell, B., Heider, J., Kaplan, B. (1966). *The Inventory of Home Stimulation.* Paper presented at the meeting of the American Psychological Association, Washington, DC.
Centers for Disease Control. (1978). *Preventing lead poisoning in young children.* Atlanta: U.S. Department of Health, Education and Welfare.
Centers for Disease Control. (1985). *Preventing lead poisoning in young children.* Atlanta: U.S. Department of Health, Education and Welfare.
Chamberlain, A.C., Heard, M.J., Little, P., Newton, D., Wells, A.C., & Wiffen, R.D. (1978). *Investigation into lead from motor vehicles.* Harwell, United Kingdom: United Kingdom Atomic Energy Authority, Report No. AERE–R9198.
Chatterjee, P., & Gettman, J.H. (1972). Lead poisoning: Subculture as a facilitating agent? *American Journal of Clinical Nutrition, 25,* 324–330.
Cravioto, J., & DeLicardie, E. (1972). Environmental correlates of severe malnutrition and language development in survivors from Kwashiorkor and Marasmus. In *Nutrition: The nervous system and behavior.* Scientific Publication No 251. Washington, DC.: Pan American Health Organization.
de la Burde, B., & Choate, M.S. (1972) Does asymptomatic lead exposure in children have latent sequelae? *Journal of Pediatrics, 81,* 1088–1091.
de la Burde, B., & Choate, M.S. (1975) Early symptomatic lead exposure and development at school age. *Journal of Pediatrics, 87,* 638–642.
Delves, H. (1970). A micro sampling method for the rapid determination of lead by atomic absorption spectrometry. *Analyst,* 95, 431–438.
Dietrich, K.N., Krafft, K.M., Pearson, D.T., Harris, L.C., Bornschein, R.L., Hammond, P.B., & Succop, P.A. (1985). The contribution of social and developmental factors to lead exposure during the first year of life. *Pediatrics, 75,* 1114–1119.
Dobbing, J. (1970). Undernutrition and the developing brain. In W.A. Hamwick (Ed.), *Developmental neurology.* Springfield, IL: Thomas.
Dolcourt, J. (1977). Lead poisoning in children of battery plant employees in North Carolina. *Morbidity and Mortality Weekly Reports.* September 30.
Dolcourt, J., Hamrick, H., O'Tuama, L., Wooten, J., & Baker, E.L. (1978). Increased lead burden in children of battery workers. *Pediatrics, 62,* 561–563.
Dunn, L.M., & Dunn, A.M. (1981). Peabody Picture Vocabulary Test, Revised. Circle Pines, MN: American Guidance Service.
Ediger, R.D., & Coleman, R.L. (1972). Modified Delves Cup atomic absorpting procedure for determination of lead in blood. *Atomic Absorpting Newsletter, 11,* 33.
Elardo, R., Bradley, R., & Caldwell, B.M. (1975). The relation of infants' home environments to mental test performance from six to thirty-six months: A longitudinal analysis. *Child Development, 46,* 71–76.
Ernhart, C.B., Landa, B., Schell, N.B. (1981). Subclinical levels of lead and development deficit-A multivariate follow-up reassessment. *Pediatrics, 67,* 911–919.
Harvey, P., Hamlin, M., Kumar, R. (1983). The Birmingham blood lead study. Paper read at the Annual Conference of the British Psychological Society, York Univ., U.K. Unpublished manuscript.
Harvey, P.G., Hamlin, M.W., Kumar, R., & Delves, H.T. (1984). Blood lead, behavior and intelligence test performance in preschool children. *The Science of the Total Environment, 40,* 45–60.
Hawk, B., & Schroeder, S.R. (1983). Factors interactive with IQ and blood lead levels in children. Paper presented at the XVIth Annual Conference on Mental Retardation and Developmental Disabilities, Gatlinburg, TN.
Hawk, B.A., Schroeder, S.R., Robinson, G., Otto, D., Mushak, P., Kleinbaum, D., & Dawson, G. (1985). Relation of lead and social factors to IQ of low SES children: A partial replication. Manuscript submitted for publication.
Heber, R. (1970). *Epidemiology of mental retardation.* Springfield, IL: Thomas.

Hollingshead, A.B. (1957). Two-factor index of social position. Unpublished manuscript. (Available from A.B. Hollingshead, 1965 Yale Station, New Haven Connecticut).

Kleinbaum, D., Kupper, L., & Morgenstern, H. (1982). *Epidemiologic research: Principles and quantitative methods.* London: Lifetime Learning Publications.

Kotok, D. (1972). Development of children with elevated blood levels: A controlled study. *Journal of Pediatrics, 80,* 57–61.

Kotok, D., Kotok, D., & Heriot, J.T. (1977). Cognitive evaluation of children with elevated blood lead levels. *American Journal of Diseases of Children, 131,* 791–793.

Landrigan, P.J., Whitworth, R.H., Baloh, R.W., Staehling, N.W., Barthel, W.F., & Rosenblum, B.F. (1975). Neuropsychological dysfunction in children with chronic low-lead absorpting. *Lancet, I,* 708–712.

Lansdown, R.G., Sheperd, J., Clayton, R.E., Delves, H.T., Graham, P.J., & Turner, W.C. (1974). Blood lead levels, behavior, and intelligence: A population study, *Lancet, I,* 538–541.

Mahaffey, K.R., & Michaelson, I.A. (1980). The interaction between lead and nutrition. In H. Needleman (Ed.), *Low level lead exposure: The clinical implications of current research* (pp. 159–200). New York: Raven Press.

McBride, W.G., Black, B.P., & English, B.J. (1982). Blood lead levels and behavior of 400 preschool children. *Medical Journal of Australia, 2,* 26–29.

McNeil, J.L., Ptasnik, J.A., & Croft, D.B. (1975). Evaluation of congestion effects of elevated blood lead concentrations in asymptomatic children. *Archives of Industrial Hygiene and Toxicology, 21,* Supplement.

Milar, C., & Mushak, P. (1982). Lead-contaminated housedust: Hazard, measurement, and decontamination. In J. Chisholm and D. O'Hara (Eds.), *Management of increased lead absorption in children: Clinical, social, and environmental aspects.* Baltimore: Urban & Schwarzenburg.

Milar, C.R., & Schroeder, S.R. (1983). The effects of lead on retardation of cognitive and adaptive behavior. In J.L. Matson and F. Andrasik (Eds.), *Treatment issues and innovations in mental retardation* (pp. 129–158). New York: Plenum Press.

Milar, C.R., Schroeder, S.R., Mushak, P., & Boone, L. (1981). Failure to find hyperactivity in preschool children with moderately elevated lead burden. *Journal of Pediatric Psychology, 6,* 85–95.

Milar, C.R., Schroeder, S.R., Mushak, P., Dolcourt, J.L., & Grant, L.D. (1980). Contributions of the caregiving environment to increased lead burden in children. *American Journal of Mental Deficiency, 84,* 339–344.

Millican, F.K., Lourie, R.S., & Layman, E.M. (1956). Emotional factors in the etiology and treatment of lead poisoning. *American Journal of Diseases of Children, 91,* 144–149.

Moore, M.R., Meredith, P.A., & Goldberg, A. (1980). Lead and hemebiosynthesis. In P.L. Singhal & J.A. Thomas (Eds.), *Lead toxicity* (pp. 79–118). Baltimore: Urban and Swarzenburg.

National Academy of Sciences. (1976). National Research Council, *Recommendation for the prevention of lead poisoning in children.* National Academy of Sciences, Washington, DC. Available from NTIS, Springfield, VA: PB257645.

National Academy of Sciences. (1980). *Lead in the human environment.* Committee on Lead in the Human Environment, National Academy of Sciences, Washington, DC.

Needleman, H.L., Gunnoe, C., Leviton, A., Reed, R., Peresie, J., Maher, C., & Barrett, B.S. (1979). Deficits in psychologic and classroom performance of children with elevated dentine levels. *New England Journal of Medicine, 13,* 689–695.

Needleman, H.L., & Landrigan, P.J. (1981). The health effects of low level exposure to lead. *Annual Review of Public Health, 2,* 277–298.

Otto, D.A., Benignus, V.A., Muller, K.E., & Barton, C.N. (1981). Effects of age and body lead burden on CNS function in young children. I. Slow cortical potentials. *EEG Clinical Neurophysiology, 52,* 229–239.

Perino, J., & Ernhart, C.B. (1974). The relation of subclinical lead level to cognitive and sensorimotor impairment in black preschoolers. *Journal of Learning Disabilities, 7,* 26–30.

Piomelli, S., Corash, L., Corash, M., Seaman, C., Mushak, P., Glover, B., & Padgett, R.

(1980). Blood lead concentrations in a remote Himalayan population. *Science, 210,* 1135–1137.

Piomelli, S., Seaman, C., Zullow, D., Curran, A., & Davidow, B. (1982). Threshold for lead damage to heme synthesis in urban children. *Proceedings of the National Academy of Sciences, 79,* 3335–3339.

Rabinowitz, M.B., Wetherill, G.W., & Kopple, J.D. (1977). Magnitude and lead intake from respiration by normal man. *Journal of Laboratory and Clinical Medicine, 90,* 238–248.

Ramey, C.T., Farran, D.C., & Campbell, F.A. (1979). Predicting IQ from mother-child interactions. *Child Development, 50,* 804–814.

Ratcliffe, J.M. (1977). Developmental and behavioral functions in young children with elevated blood lead levels. *British Journal of Preventive Social Medicine, 31,* 258–264.

Read, M.S. (1982). Malnutrition and behavior. *Applied Research in Mental Retardation, 3,* 279–291.

Rennert, O.M., Weiner, P., & Madden, J. (1970). Asymptomatic lead poisoning in 85 Chicago children. *Clinical Pediatrics, 9,* 9–13.

Rummo, J.H. (1974). Intellectual and behavioral effects of lead poisoning in children. Unpublished doctoral dissertation, University of North Carolina.

Rummo, J.H., Routh, D.K., Rummo, H.J., & Brown, J.F. (1979). Behavioral and neurological effects of symptomatic and asymptomatic lead exposure in children. *Archives of Environmental Health, 34,* 120–124.

Sameroff, A.J., & Chandler, M.J. (1975). Reproductive risk and the continuum of caretaking casualty. In F.D. Horowitz (Ed.), *Review of Child Development Research (Vol. 4)* (pp. 187–244). Chicago: The University of Chicago Press.

Schroeder, S., Hawk, B., Otto, D., Mushak, P., & Hicks, R. (1985). Separating the effects of lead and social factors on IQ. *Environmental Research, 38,* 144–154.

Smith, M., Delves, T., Lansdown, R., Clayton, B., & Graham, P. (1983). The effects of lead exposure on urban children: The Institute of Child Health/Southampton Study. *Developmental Medicine and Child Neurology, 26,* Supplement No. 6.

Snowdon, C.F. (1977). A nutritional basis for lead pica. *Physiology and Behavior, 18,* 888–893.

U.S. Environmental Protection Agency. (1977). Air Quality for Lead. EPA–600/8–77–017. Washington, DC.

U.S. Environmental Protection Agency (1986). Air Quality Criteria for Lead, Vol. IV, EPA–600/8–83–028A. Washington, DC.

Weiss, B. (1980). Conceptual issues in the assessment of lead toxicity. In H. Needleman (Ed.), *Low level lead exposure: The clinical implications of current research.* New York: Raven Press.

Werner, E., Honzik, M., & Smith, R. (1968). Prediction of intelligence and achievement at ten years from twenty months, pediatric and psychological examinations. *Child Development, 39,* 1063–1075.

White, K.R. (1982). The relation between socioeconomic status and academic achievement. *Psychological Bulletin, 91*(3), 461–481.

White, B., & Watts, J.C. (1973). *Experience and environment: Major influences on the development of the young child.* Englewood Cliffs, NJ: Prentice-Hall.

Winneke, G., Hrdina, K.G., & Brockhaus, A. (1982). Neuropsychological studies in children with elevated tooth-lead concentration. Part I: Pilot study. *International Archives of Occupational Environmental Health, 51,* 169–183.

Winneke, G., Kramer, U., Brockhaus, A., Ewers, U., Kujanek, G., Lechner, H., & Janke, W. (1983). Neuropsychological studies in children with elevated tooth-lead concentrations. Part II: Extended study. *International Archives of Occupational Environmental Health, 51,* 231–252.

Winneke, G., & Kraemer, U. (1984). Neuropsychological effects of lead in children: Interactions with social background variables. *Neuropsychobiology, 11,* 195–202.

Yule, W., Lansdown, R., Millar, I.B., & Urbanowicz, M.A. (1981). The relationship between blood lead concentrations, intelligence and attainment in a school population: A pilot study. *Developmental Medicine and Child Neurology, 23,* 567–576.

Yule, W., & Lansdown, R. (1983). Lead and children's development: Recent findings. In *Proceedings of Heidelberg Conference on heavy metals in the environment.* Heidelberg, FRG.

Yule, W., Lansdown, R., Hunter, J., Urbanowicz, M.A., Clayton, B., & Delves, I. (1983). Blood lead concentrations in school age children: Intelligence, attainment, and behaviour. Paper presented at the Annual Conference of the British Psychological Society, York, England, April.

Yule, W., Urbanowicz, M.A., Lansdown, R., & Millar, I.B. (1984). Teachers' ratings of children's behavior in relation to blood lead levels. *British Journal of Developmental Psychology, 2,* 295–305.

Ziegler, E.E., Edwards, B.B., Jensen, R.C., Mahaffey, K.R., & Fomon, S.J. (1978). Absorption and retention of lead by infants. *Pediatric Research, 12,* 29–34.

The Assessment of Neurotoxicity in Children

Electrophysiological Methods[1]

David A. Otto
U.S. Environmental Protection Agency

Neurotoxicity assessment in young children poses a considerable challenge because of language and behavioral constraints. Traditional psychophysical threshold, psychomotor, and cognitive tasks used in behavioral toxicology cannot reliably be administered to children below 3 to 5 years of age. On the other hand, this subset of the population is uniquely susceptible to neurotoxic impairment because of the immaturity of the nervous system. Development of an electrophysiological assessment battery that is free of linguistic and motor constraints would thus provide a useful contribution for neurotoxicity testing in young children.

Criteria to be considered in selecting pediatric neurotoxicity measures are listed in Table 1. Neurotoxicity tests should meet the selection criteria required of psychometric tests—that is, each test should be standardized, valid, reliable, and objective. Most importantly, tests must be sensitive to the effects of toxicant exposure. Tests should also be noninvasive and nonthreatening, culture free, and as age independent as possible. Standard psychometric tests (e.g., IQ tests) are age dependent and widely criticized as culturally biased. If the objective is population screening (as opposed to clinical evaluation), three additional criteria should be considered in test selection. Tests should be rapid (as a rule of thumb, the battery should be limited to about 30 minutes in length), simple to administer and score, and inexpensive.

Are there electrophysiological measures that meet these stringent criteria? Peripheral nerve conduction velocity (NCV) is the most widely used electrophysiological measure in human neurotoxicity testing. However, there is substantial doubt regarding the sensitivity of NCV measures in young children because of the wide range of normal variability. Other evoked brain potential measures have been clinically

---

[1] The research described in this article has been reviewed by the Health Effects Research Laboratory, U.S. Environmental Protection Agency, and approved for publication. Approval does not signify that the contents necessarily reflect the views and policies of the Agency.

TABLE 1

Selection Criteria for Pediatric Neurotoxicity Tests

Criterion	Description
1. Nonverbal	Test does not require verbal instruction or verbal response
2. Nonmotoric	Test does not require any voluntary motor response
3. Noninvasive	Test does not require skin penetration
4. Nonthreatening	Test does not frighten or upset children
5. Age independent	Test scores vary minimally with age
6. Culture free	Test scores do not vary with ethnic background or social class
7. Standardized	Standard procedures for test administration and measurement have been developed, published, and accepted by user community; normative data available for evaluation of clinical significance of data
8. Valid	Test measures the dimension or function that it was selected to assess
9. Reliable	Test provides comparable results when administered on repeated occasions
10. Sensitive	Test discriminates between exposed and nonexposed populations; detects change at minimal effect threshold
11. Objective	Test provides a quantitative measure that is not susceptible to subjective measurement bias
12. Rapid	For population testing, individual measures should require no more than 10 minutes to administer; rapid scoring of response is also important
13. Simple	Test should be simple to administer, simple for the subject to perform, and simple to score
14. Inexpensive	Cost of test materials, administration, and scoring within reasonable limits

validated for the assessment of auditory, visual, and somatosensory function in the central nervous system. These tests—including the *brainstem auditory* (BAEP), *pattern-reversal visual* (PREP), and *somatosensory* (SEP) *evoked potentials*—require no motor expression and minimal language comprehension. Each has achieved widespread clinical application during the past decade in the assessment of sensory pathway integrity and nonspecific demyelinating diseases such as multiple sclerosis (Aminoff, 1980; Desmedt, 1980; Starr, Sohmer, & Celesia, 1978).

Otto (1983) and Arezzo, Simson, and Brennan (1985) have reviewed the use of evoked potentials in occupational medicine and human neurotoxicity assessment. BAEPs, PREPs, and SEPs have seldom been used for neurotoxicity testing in children and only meager evidence has been obtained in adults. Seppalainen (1978) compared the sensitivity of NCV and SEP as indices of subclinical neuropathy in lead workers. She reported that the SEP detected impairments at lower blood lead levels than did NCV measures. Seppalainen, Raitta, and Huuskonen (1980) used visual evoked potentials (VEP) in a study of workers exposed to n-hexane. VEP deficits were noted in 14 of 15 workers studied. VEPs are elicited by diffuse photic stimulation, while PREPs are elicited by a reversing checkerboard. PREPs are more sensitive than VEPs in diagnosing optic nerve degeneration and multiple sclerosis (Halliday, McDonald, & Mushin, 1972, 1973). Pattern-reversal EPs may, therefore, be more sensitive than flash EPs to toxicant substances that affect visual function.

BRAINSTEM AUDITORY EVOKED POTENTIAL

Figure 1 illustrates a typical BAEP. Note the time scale. Seven components occur within 10 msec of click onset. Successive components reflect the transmission of the afferent signal from the acoustic nerve to the thalamus, each component reflecting a relay in the auditory pathway. Although the precise origins of these components are still debated (e.g., Scherg & Von Cramon, 1985), enough is known to accurately localize lesions in the auditory pathway. The variability of component latencies, particularly components I, III, and V, is so small that a slight increase in component latency is indicative of pathology in the auditory pathway. Simple measures permit determination of central or peripheral levels of

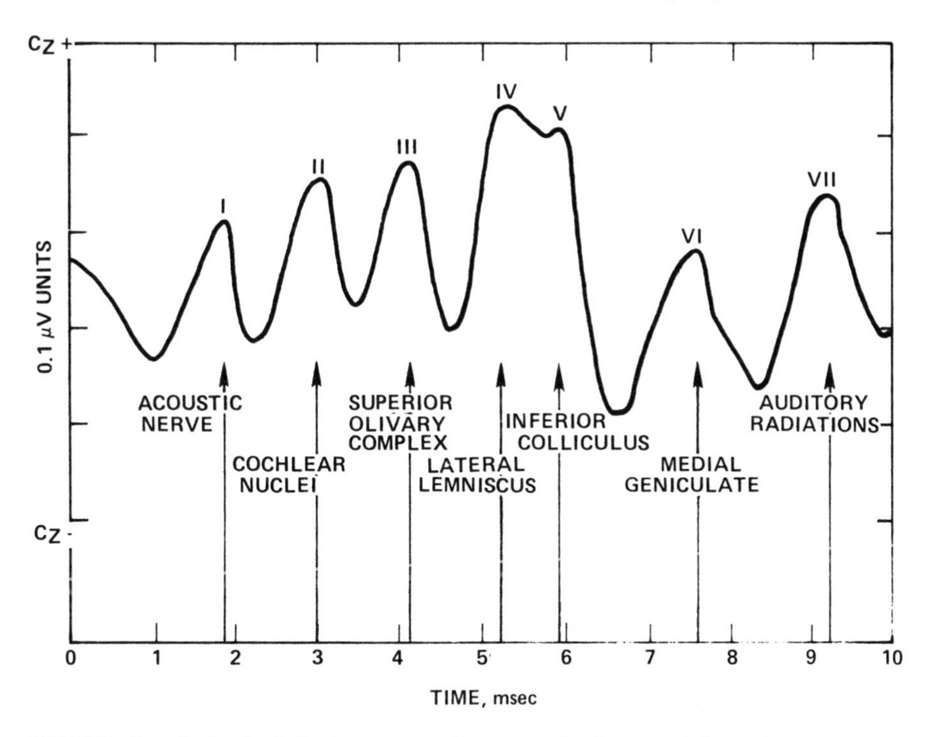

FIGURE 1. A typical brainstem auditory evoked potential with presumed origins of successive components.

damage. Because the amplitude of BAEP components is usually less than 0.5 μV, a million-fold amplification and large number (2000–4000) of trials may be necessary to obtain adequate signal-to-noise resolution. Click stimuli can be presented rapidly (up to 50 Hz), however, so that an average may require less than 1 minute. For screening purposes, a click rate of about 30 Hz is recommended (Schwartz & Berry, 1985).

The BAEP is remarkably robust and is not affected by arousal level—for instance, a normal BAEP can be recorded in a comatose patient as long as the auditory pathway is intact (Starr, 1977). Clinicians, in fact, prefer to record BAEPs in *sleeping* children to avoid an electromyographic (EMG) artifact that accompanies movement (Jerger, Hayes, & Jordan, 1980). Trials containing an EMG artifact must be rejected, making it difficult to record from uncooperative children. In clinical practice sedatives are usually administered to young children prior to recording BAEPs. We have found that most children can be coaxed to relax or fall asleep for BAEP testing without sedation (Otto et al., 1985).

Figure 2 illustrates a useful maturational feature of the BAEP. Adult latencies are reached by the age of 18 months. BAEPs thus offer measures of peripheral and central auditory function that are practically age independent.

Evidence from studies of children with undue lead absorption (Otto et al., 1985; Robinson, Baumann, Schroeder, Mushak, & Otto, 1985) suggests, furthermore, that BAEPs are sensitive to heavy metal exposure. Latencies of peaks III and V (Otto et al., 1985) and interpeak latency V-I (Robinson et al., 1985) increased directly with blood lead levels as illustrated in Figure 3.

PATTERN-REVERSAL VISUAL EVOKED POTENTIAL

Figure 4 illustrates a typical PREP. This waveform is elicited by a reversing checkerboard pattern in which dark and light squares alternate to maintain constant luminance levels. The PREP reflects activity primarily from the fovea (central three degrees of the visual field) because: (a) foveal cells project to the surface of the visual cortex, while peripheral retinal cells project to areas deep within the calcarine fissure; and (b) foveal representation in the cortex is disproportionately greater than peripheral visual projections (Sokol, 1980). The latency of the P100 component is sensitive to visual pathway lesions. Increased latencies indicative of optic neuritis or multiple sclerosis can be reliably detected prior to the emergence of clinical symptoms (Halliday et al., 1972, 1973). Because many neurotoxicants affect visual function (see Table 2), the PREP is a recommended component of a neurotoxicity test battery.

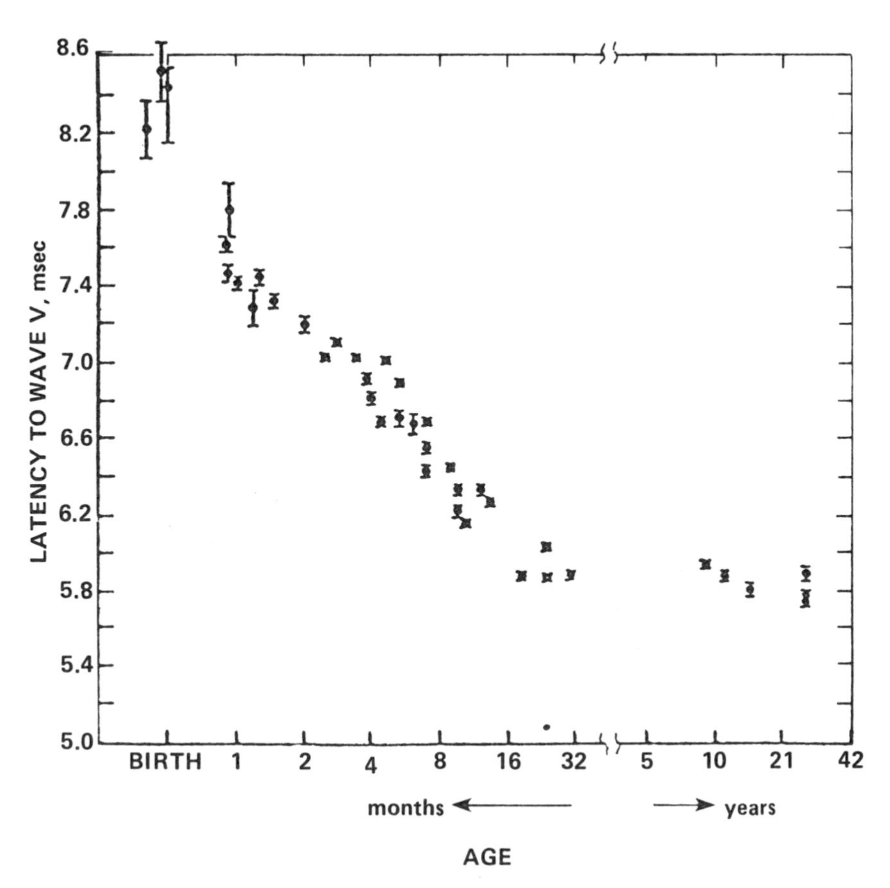

FIGURE 2. Latency of wave V response to 60 dB SL click as a function of age. A systematic decrease in latency occurs from birth to about 18 months of age. Each point represents an average of at least three measurements for individual subjects. (Redrawn from Hecox and Galambos, 1974.)

Important features of the PREP waveform vary systematically with stimulus intensity, check size, presentation rate, retinal locus of stimulation, and quality of the display. Detailed consideration of these methodological factors is beyond the scope of the present discussion, but excellent reviews are available (Desmedt, 1977; Sokol, 1976, 1980). To summarize briefly, P100 amplitude decreases and latency increases as pattern intensity (luminance) or optical quality decreases. Smaller checks tend to elicit more complex waveforms than larger checks at slow presentation rates. A transition from a multi-peak to a single-peak waveform (called a *steady state potential*) occurs at alternation rates between

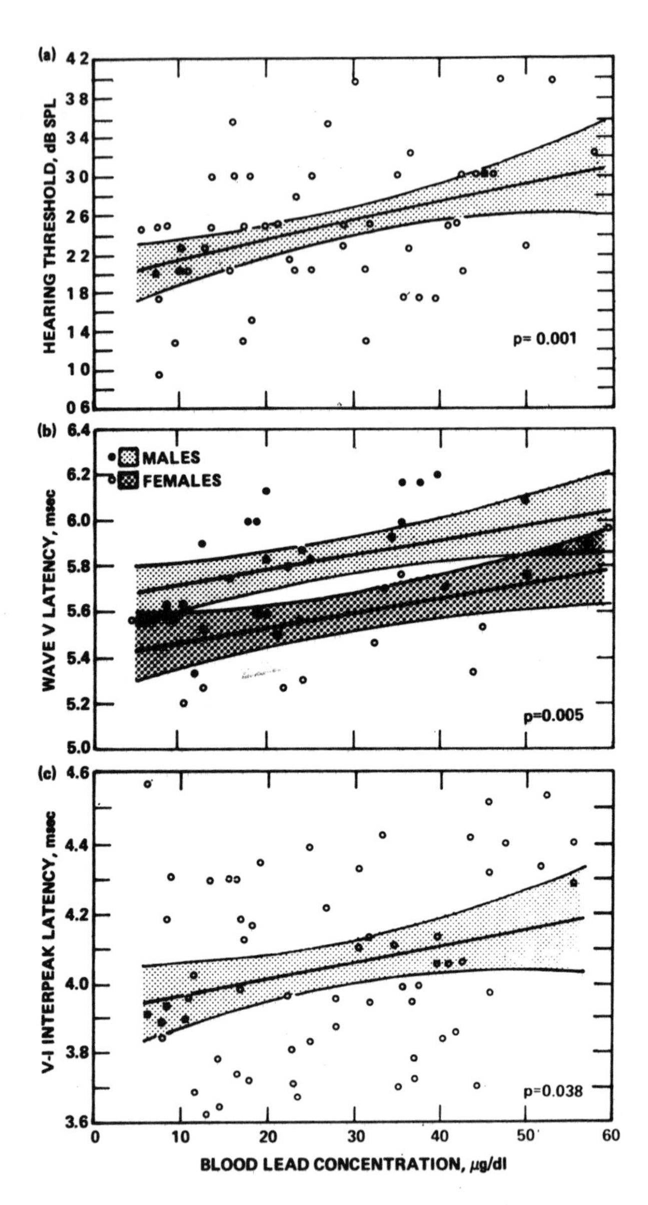

FIGURE 3. Scatter plots, regression lines, and 95% confidence limits of (a) hearing threshold (Robinson et al., 1985), (b) BAEP wave latencies of boys and girls (Otto et al., 1985), and (c) BAEP interpeak V-I latencies of children (Robinson et al., 1985) as functions of blood lead levels. Hearing thresholds were determined audiometrically using a 2 KHz pure tone. Linear increases in hearing threshold, latencies of BAEP waves III and IV, and V-I interpeak latency were observed with increasing blood lead concentrations.

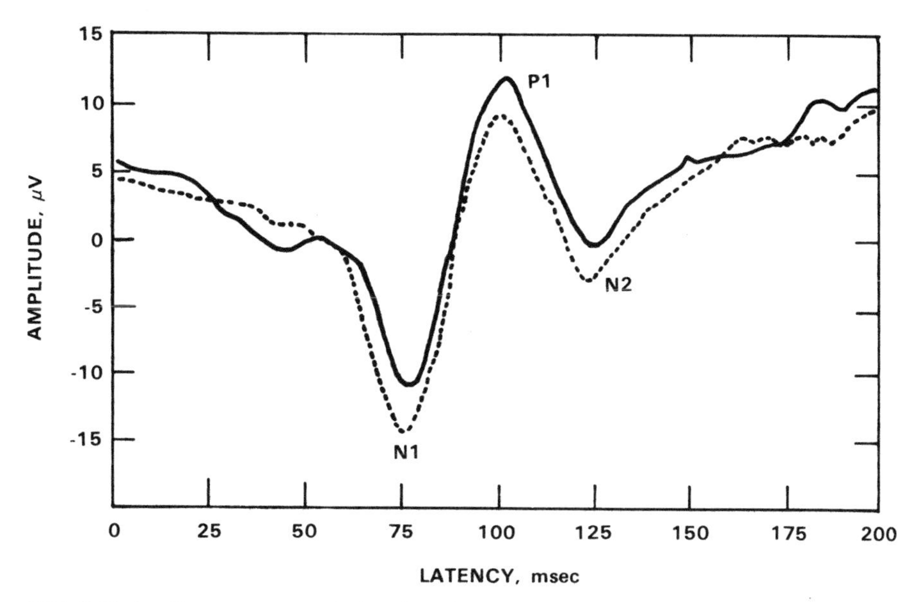

FIGURE 4. Pattern-reversal visual evoked potentials recorded from a 6-year-old boy. Replicate waveforms were obtained using binocular stimulation from black and white squares subtending 24° visual angle, 90% contrast, and reversing twice per sec. Latencies of N1, P1, and N2 components and N1P1 amplitude were measured.

6 and 10 per second, depending on check size (Figure 5). Because the PREP reflects cone activation, selective parafoveal stimulation does not elicit a clearly defined waveform.

Several subject parameters, including pupil size and level of light adaptation, also affect P100 amplitude and latency. Pupil size controls retinal luminance. In particular, clinical disorders such as glaucoma, medications, or adaptation levels that produce miosis (pupil constriction) depress amplitude and increase latency of the P100 component. It is thus important to check pupil diameter at the time of testing; the test should not be run if pupils are miotic or dilated. For neurotoxicity testing, the stimulus parameters noted above, pupil diameter, and the level of light adaptation must be rigorously standardized across subjects.

P100 latency also varies with age, an important factor in assessing pediatric populations. Sokol and Jones (1979) have shown that P100 latency decreases rapidly during the first year of life and then slowly until about 5 years of age (Figure 6). The latency x age function varies also with check size; P100 latency matures earlier for large checks than small checks.

TABLE 2

Substances Toxic to the Visual System in Humans

Absinthe	Lindane
Antirabies	Mercuric chloride
Arsenicals (organic)	Methanol
Bee sting	Methyl acetate
Carbon dioxide	Methyl bromide
Carbon disulfide	DL-Penicillamine
Carbon monoxide	Phosphorus
Carbon tetrachloride	Quinine
Cassava	Snake venoms
Clioquinol	Streptomycin
Cobalt chloride	Tetraethyl lead
Cyanide	Thallium
Dinitrotoluene	Tobacco smoke
Disulfiram	Trichlorethylene
Ergot	Trinitrobenzene
Ethylene glycol	Trinitrotoluene
Hexachlorophene	Vincristine
Lead	Wasp sting

Note. Evidence indicates that these substances affect either intraretinal neurons or optic fibers (Grant, 1980).

Little change in P100 latency occurs after 6 months of age for check sizes 30 minutes of arc or larger.

PREP testing of young children is difficult because it is neccessary to fixate on a reversing checkerboard for several minutes. Each average requires 100–200 reversals at a rate of about 2 per second. At least two averages should be obtained for each test to assure reliability. If each eye were tested separately, the complete test would require about 8 minutes of fixation, assuming the use of a single check size and single stimulus rate.

Young children do not tolerate eye patches well. Monocular recordings in young children are thus difficult to obtain. Because lead (and other neurotoxicants) produce diffuse, nonspecific effects on CNS function, our PREP protocol included two binocular tests only. Inconsistent findings in two samples of children at risk for lead poisoning (Otto et al., 1985; Otto, in press), however, indicate the need for further study to determine the optimal stimulus parameters for neurotoxicity testing.

If toxicant exposure impairs scotopic (rod-mediated) vision more than photopic (cone-mediated) vision, the PREP waveform is unlikely to be affected, since it reflects cone activation. Lead and carbon monoxide (McFarland, Roughton, Halperin, & Niven, 1944; Sillman, Bolnick, Bosetti, Haynes, & Walter, 1982) both seem to show more pronounced effects under dark adapted (scoptic) conditions. Flash evoked potentials

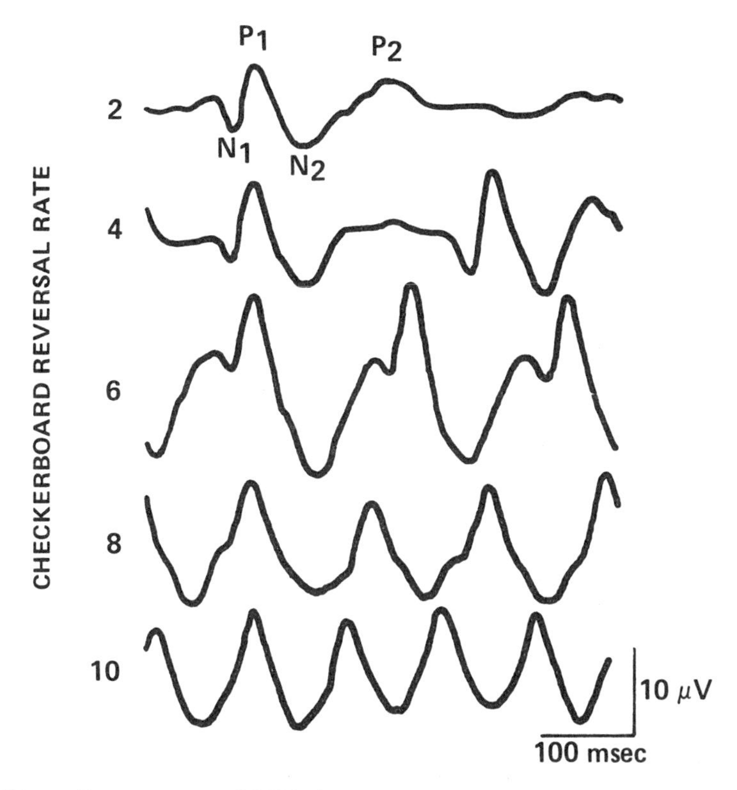

FIGURE 5. Pattern reversal VEPs in response to 12-minute checks for different alternation rates. Alternation rate per second is shown to the left of the records. Note the change from transient to steady state VEPs between 6 and 10 reversals per second. (Redrawn from Sokol, 1980.)

(Wooten, 1972) or contrast sensitivity (Arden, 1979) methods may provide better visual function tests in these cases.

ASSESSMENT OF SOMATOSENSORY FUNCTION

In some respects the somatosensory system is ideal for neurotoxicity testing. Somatosensory pathways, stretching from the hands and feet to the cortex, are extremely long and can be assessed with noninvasive electrophysiological methods as different levels of synaptic transmission. Peripheral nerve conduction velocity (NCV) has long been used by neurologists to diagnose peripheral neuropathy in workers exposed to lead and other toxic chemicals (Seppalainen, 1975). Arrival of the afferent

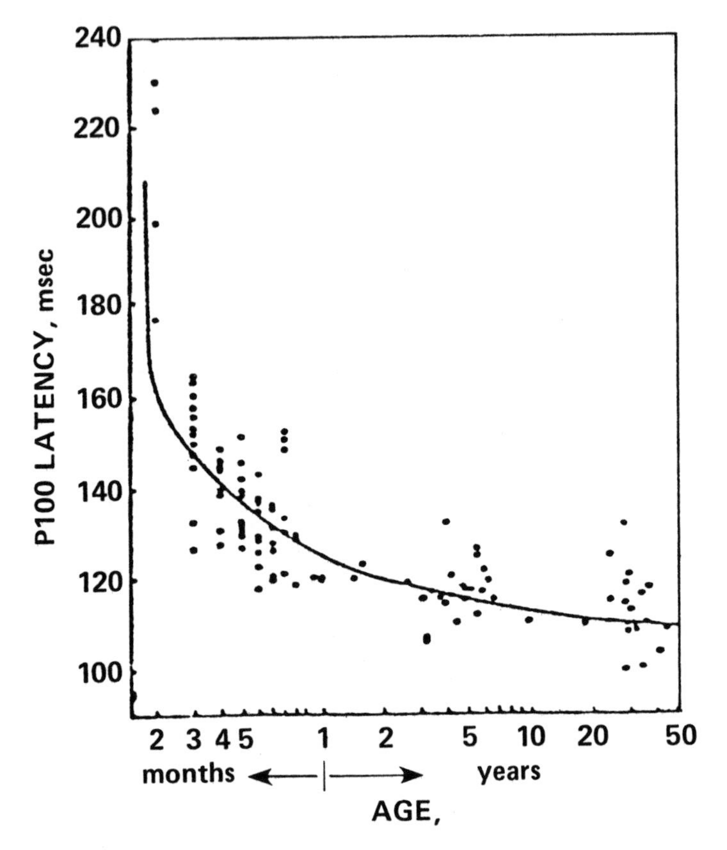

FIGURE 6. Latency of P100 component for 15′ checks as a function of age from infancy to adulthood. The curve was derived by least squares fit. (Redrawn from Sokol and Jones, 1979.)

signal in somatosensory cortex can also be recorded from scalp electrodes using signal averaging procedures. Newer evoked potential techniques have been developed to assess neurological disorders in the spinal cord, brainstem, and thalamus (Noel & Desmedt, 1980).

Despite widespread use of somatosensory evoked potentials (SEPs) in clinical neurology, little effort has been made to apply SEPs in human neurotoxicity assessment. Seppalainen (1978) reported that the scalp-recorded SEP was more sensitive than NCV as an index of subclinical neuropathy in lead exposed workers. Arezzo, Schaumburg, Vaughan, Spencer, and Barna (1982) reported that SEP changes precede behavioral or NCV alterations in monkeys exposed to acrylamide. Schaumburg, Arezzo, Markowitz & Spencer (1981) noted some problems that confront the application of SEPs in human neurotoxicity testing: waveforms vary with age, skin temperature, body size, and location of scalp electrodes. The noxious nature of electric stimuli may be problematic in pediatric testing. The potential versatility and sensitivity of the SEP, however, argue for inclusion of this measure in a general neurotoxicity screening battery.

Figure 7 illustrates a method described by Eisen and Odusote (1980) of measuring central and peripheral conduction time following median nerve stimulation. Surface electrodes are placed at several convenient anatomical landmarks that permit the derivation of central and peripheral components. The stimulating electrode (S) is attached at the wrist over the median nerve. Peripheral conduction time between the wrist and brachial

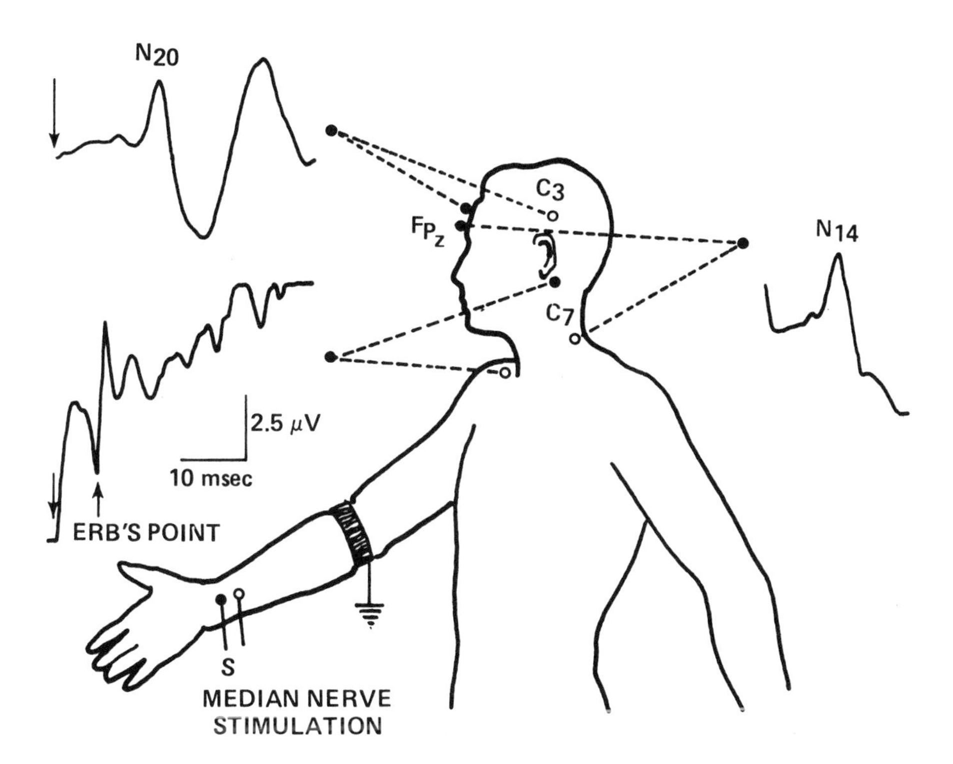

FIGURE 7. Procedure to derive central and peripheral conduction times in somatosensory pathways following median nerve stimulation. (Adapted from Eisen and Odusote, 1980.)

plexus is obtained by recording from an electrode at Erb's point in the supraclavicular fossa referred to the mastoid process. The initial component of the Erb's point potential reflects the arrival of the afferent volley in the brachial plexus. Peripheral conduction time recorded in this manner from normal, healthy adults is 8.9 ± 0.7 msec.

Central conduction time from dorsal column nuclei to cortex is derived from two other measures. Arrival of the sensory volley in the dorsal column nuclei is reflected in the N14 component of the cervical SEP. The cervical SEP is recorded from an electrode (C7) placed at the base of the neck between the 6th and 7th cervical spines. C7 is referenced to a midfrontal (Fpz) lead. Arrival of the afferent volley at the cortex is reflected in the N20 component of the SEP recorded over contralateral somatosensory cortex (C3 or C4) referred to Fpz. Central conduction time from dorsal column nuclei to cortex is calculated as the difference (N20−N14) between the cortical and cervical components. The value obtained by Eisen and Odusote (1980) from normal, healthy adults is 5.1 ± 0.6 msec.

The maturation of the somatosensory evoked potential has been studied by Desmedt, Brunko, and Debecker (1976, 1980). These investigators described the developmental course of the N22 component evoked by finger stimulation. This component is analogous to the N20 component elicited by median nerve stimulation. The developmental pattern, illustrated in Figure 8, is complicated by the fact that peripheral and central segments of the lengthy pathway mature at different rates and the fact that SEP latency depends on body size (nerve length), which varies greatly during development. Body size and N22 latency normalized for body size are plotted in Figure 8, lower section. The normalized latency decreases sharply during the first 18 months, then decreases slowly to about 8 years of age. Peripheral afferent axons mature rapidly during the first year (Gamstorp & Shelburne, 1965). Figure 8, upper section, exhibits the constancy of N22 onset latency from 6 months to 8 years. Considerable work is needed to establish the maturational course of SEP components recorded at different synaptic levels of the somatosensory pathway.

EVENT-RELATED SLOW POTENTIALS

In addition to sensory evoked potentials, there is another family of electrophysiological measures related to information processing, cognition, and memory. These waveforms are collectively called *event-related slow potentials* (ERSPs) or *association potentials*. The three most prominent ERSPs are: (a) contingent negative variation (CNV)—a slow vertex-

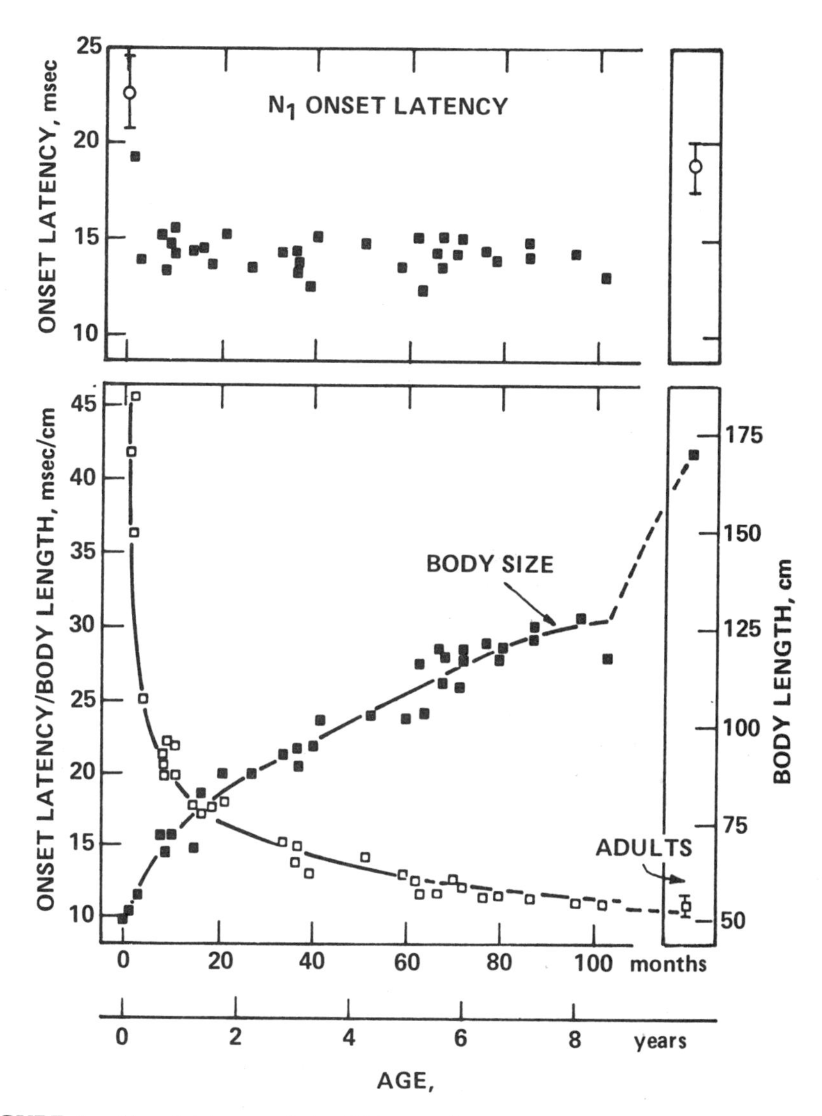

FIGURE 8. Onset latency of the N22 negative cortical component as a function of postnatal maturation in normal children in the waking state. Upper section: Data from 39 newborns in REM sleep appear as a single point to the left abscissa zero. Each data point represents an average of at least 3 SEPs from an individual child. Data from 16 normal adults appear on the right (mean and SD). Onset latency of N22 in msec. Lower section: body length (cm) with the corresponding scale on the right and onset latency of N22 divided by body length (msec/cm) with the corresponding scale on the left. (From Desmedt et al., 1976.)

negative shift in scalp-recorded EEG that arises during a signalled reaction time foreperiod (Walter, Cooper, Aldridge, McCallum, & Winter, 1964); (b) readiness potential (RP)—a slow vertex-negative shift in EEG baseline that arises about 1 second prior to a stereotyped movement (Kornhuber & Deecke, 1965); and (c) P300—a large positive wave that peaks 300–900 msec following a stimulus that delivers relevant information to the perceiver (Sutton, Braren, & Zubin, 1965). Preliminary efforts to apply ERSP methods in environmental toxicology have been reviewed by Otto and Reiter (1978). Groll-Knapp, Wagner, Hauck, and Haider (1972) reported a dose-related decrease in CNV amplitude in subjects exposed to low concentrations of carbon monoxide, although the same laboratory (Groll-Knapp, Haider, Hoeller, Jenker, & Stidl, 1978) was unable to replicate these results. Otto, Benignus & Prah (1978) reported a paradoxical increase in CNV amplitude in subjects exposed to 100 ppm CO, but a decrease in subjects exposed to 200 ppm CO.

The sensitivity of ERSPs to neurotoxicant exposure in children has been demonstrated in a series of studies (Otto, Benignus, Muller, & Barton, 1981; Otto, Benignus, Muller, Barton, & Schroeder, 1982; Otto et al., 1985). A linear relationship between slow wave voltage and blood lead level (Figure 9) was observed in young children during passive sensory conditioning (Otto et al., 1981). Slow wave voltage varied systematically across the observed range of blood lead levels (6–59 μg/dl)—evidence that Pb exposure alters CNS function at levels below the 25 μg/dl limit currently considered to be "safe" (Centers for Disease Control (CDC), 1985). The same relationship between slow wave voltage and PbB was observed in a 2-year follow-up (Otto et al., 1982), but not in a 5-year follow-up study (Otto et al., 1985) of the same group of children.

In the latter study, however, a linear increase in slow wave negativity with increasing lead exposure history was found (Figure 10) when a motor response requirement was added to the sensory conditioning test. Larger slow brain potentials were obtained during active than during passive testing. The active test also seems to be more sensitive than the passive test to toxicant exposure, although it cannot be used in children below the age of 4 or 5 years. See Otto (in press) for further discussion of this problem.

While the pediatric lead studies provide encouraging evidence of the utility of ERSP measures in environmental toxicology, ERSPs must still be considered experimental measures. Although the relationships among ERSPs, behavior, and cognitive processes have been exhaustively explored during the past decade (McCallum & Knott, 1973, 1976; Callaway, Tueting, & Koslow, 1978; Otto, 1978; Kornhuber & Deecke, 1980), very little is known about the anatomical, physiological, or chemical substrate of these waveforms. Even the psychological and behavioral

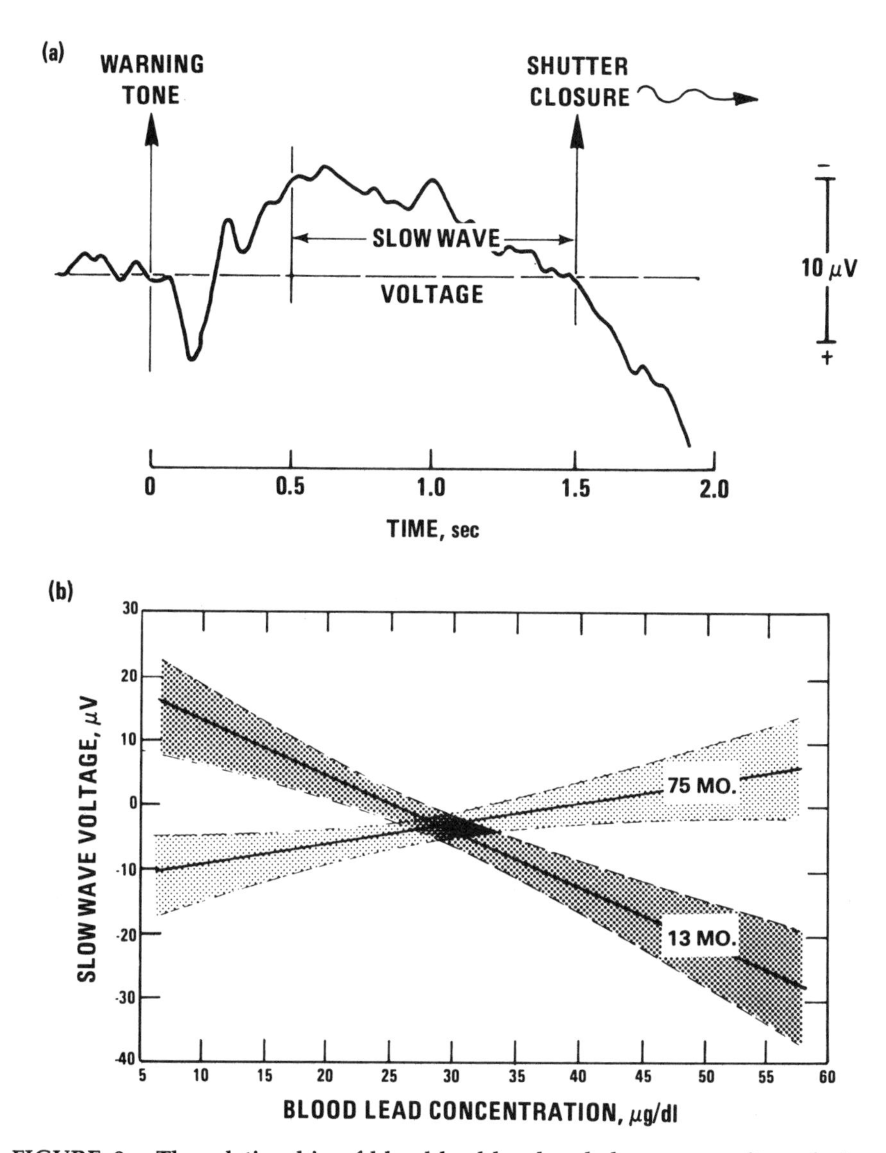

FIGURE 9. The relationship of blood lead level and slow wave voltage during passive sensory conditioning: (a) Summary average of slow potentials recorded from the vertex of children aged 1 to 6 years. Mean voltage of the slow wave during a 1 sec epoch preceding shutter closure was computed. (b) Interactive effects of age and blood lead levels on slow wave voltage. Predicted slow wave voltage and 95% confidence limits are depicted as a function of original blood lead levels at the extreme ages of subjects. (Adapted from Otto et al., 1981.)

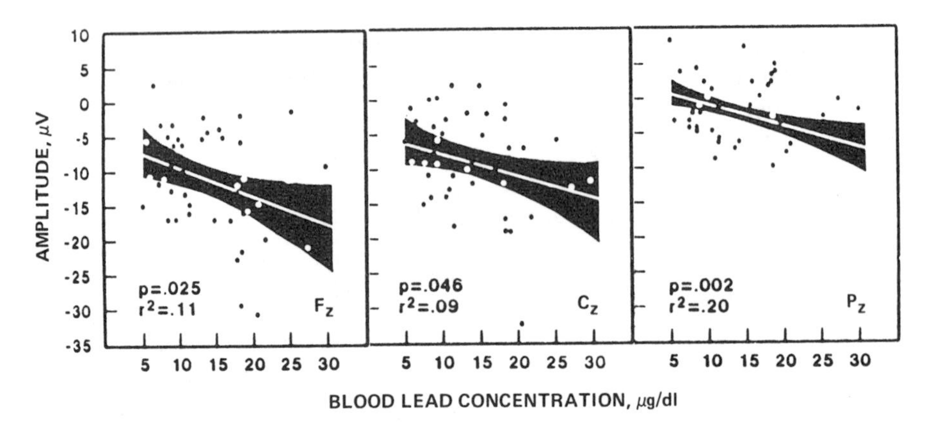

FIGURE 10. Slow potential amplitude at frontal (Fz), central (Cz), and parietal (Pz) scalp locations recorded during active sensory conditioning and plotted as a function of blood lead (PbB) levels of children on the day of testing. Slow wave negativity increased linearly with current PbB at all recording sites. Mean slow potential voltage during the half-second preceding the imperative stimulus was measured. Scatter plots of data from individual subjects are shown with 95% confidence intervals for derived regression lines. (Redrawn from Otto et al., 1985.)

significance of ERSPs remains a subject of lively controversy. Little effort has been made to standardize testing procedures or to construct population norms for any ERSP measures. Most CNV tests employ a motor response such as key pressing, while the most popular P300 test requires counting—factors that limit the use of these measures in young children.

Other methodological problems limit the application of ERSP methods in environmental toxicology, particularly in the assessment of young children. Eye and body movements produce artifacts during ERSP recording. Trials in which eye or body movements occur must be rejected from signal averages. Eye fixation on the stimulus generator is usually required to minimize eye movement artifact. The use of video cartoons to maintain eye fixation and cooperation of children has proven successful with children 30 months and older (Otto, Benignus, Seiple, Loiselle, & Hatcher, 1980), but ERSP testing of children aged 6–30 months of age remains problematic.

CONCLUSIONS

Salient features and limitations of several sensory evoked potentials that are widely used in clinical neurology and event-related slow potentials that are promising experimental measures have been described. To compare the relative merits of different electrophysiological measures as components of a pediatric neurotoxicity testing battery, each has been evaluated using the criteria specified at the outset. Table 3 indicates the ratings assigned to each measure with IQ included for comparison: a plus (+) indicates that the measure meets the selection criteria; a minus (−) indicates that the measure does not; a question mark (?) indicates that insufficient evidence is available to assign a rating. While this binary rating scheme is crude and little evidence exists to evaluate the sensitivity or utility of these tests in pediatric populations exposed to environmental toxicants, Table 3 provides a systematic basis on which to select appropriate electrophysiological measures for neurotoxicity assessment. Clinically validated tests (BAEP, PREP, and SEP) of sensory dysfunction and nonspecifc demyelinating diseases must be considered prime candidates. Event-related slow potentials including the CNV and P300 have considerable promise, but require modification, standardization, and validation to satisfy the selection criteria for a pediatric neurotoxicity test battery.

TABLE 3

Selection Criteria for Pediatric Neurotoxicity Tests

	IQ	BAEP	PREP	SEP	SW	CNV	P300
(1) Nonverbal	−	+	+	+	+	−	?
(2) Nonmotoric	−	+	+	+	+	−	+
(3) Noninvasive	+	+	+	+	+	+	+
(4) Nonthreatening	+	+	+	−	+	+	+
(5) Age independent	−	+	+	+	−	−	−
(6) Culture free	−	+	+	+	+	?	?
(7) Standardized	+	+	+	+	−	−	−
(8) Valid	+	+	+	+	?	?	?
(9) Reliable	+	+	+	+	?	?	?
(10) Sensitive	−	+	?	?	+	?	?
(11) Objective	+	+	+	+	+	+	+
(12) Rapid	−	+	+	+	−	+	+
(13) Simple	−	+	+	−	−	+	+
(14) Inexpensive	+	−	−	−	−	−	−

REFERENCES

Aminoff, M.J. (Ed.). (1980). *Electrodiagnosis in clinical neurology*. New York: Churchill Livingstone.

Arden, G.B. (1979). Measuring contrast sensitivity with gratings: A new simple technique for the early diagnosis of retinal and neurological disease. *Journal of the American Optometry Association, 50*, 35–39.

Arezzo, J., Schaumburg, H., Vaughan, H., Spencer, P., & Barna, J. (1982). Hindlimb somatosensory evoked potentials in the monkey: The effects of distal axonopathy. *Annals of Neurology, 12,* 24–32.

Arezzo, J.C., Simson, R., & Brennan, N.E. (1985). Evoked potentials in the assessment of neurotoxicity in humans. *Neurobehavioral Toxicology and Teratology, 7,* 299–304.

Callaway, E., Teuting, P., & Koslow, S. (Eds.). (1978). *Event-related brain potentials in man.* New York: Academic Press.

Centers for Disease Control. (1985). *Preventing lead poisoning in young children: A statement by the Centers for Disease Control.* Atlanta.

Desmedt, J.E. (Ed.). (1977). *Visual evoked potentials in man: New developments.* Oxford: Clarendon Press.

Desmedt, J.E. (Ed.). (1980). *Clinical uses of cerebral, brainstem, and spinal somatosensory evoked potentials. Progress in clinical neurophysiology* (Vol. 10). New York: Karger.

Desmedt, J., Brunko, E., & Debecker, J. (1976). Maturation of the somatosensory evoked potentials in normal infants and children, with particular reference to the early N1 component. *Electroencephalography and Clinical Neurophysiology, 40,* 43–58.

Desmedt, J., Brunko, E., & Debecker, J. (1980). Maturation and sleep correlates of the somatosensory evoked potential. *Progress in Clinical Neurophysiology, 7,* 147–161.

Eisen, A., & Odusote, K. (1980). Central and peripheral conduction times in multiple sclerosis. *Electroencephalography and Clinical Neurophysiology, 48,* 253–265.

Gamstorp, I., & Shelburne, A. (1965). Peripheral sensory conduction in ulnar and median nerves of normal infants, children and adolescents. *Acta Paediactrica Scandinavica, 54,* 209–313.

Grant, W.M. (1980). The peripheral vision system as a target. In P.S. Spencer & H.H. Schaumburg (Eds.), *Experimental and clinical neurotoxicity* (pp. 77–91). Baltimore: Williams and Wilkins.

Groll-Knapp, E., Haider, M., Hoeller, H., Jenker, H., & Stidl, H. (1978). Neuro- and psychophysiological effects of moderate carbon monoxide exposure. In D. Otto (Ed.), *Multidisciplinary perspectives in event-related brain potential research* (pp. 424–436). Publication No. EPA-600/9-77-043. Washington, DC: Government Printing Office.

Groll-Knapp, E., Wagner, H., Hauck, H., & Haider, M. (1972). Effects of low carbon monoxide concentrations on vigilance and computer-analyzed brain potentials. *Staub-Reinholtung Luft, 32,* 64–68.

Halliday, A.M., McDonald, W., & Mushin, J. (1972). Delayed visual evoked response in optic neuritis. *Lancet, 1,* 982–985.

Halliday, A.M., McDonald, W., & Mushin, J. (1973). Visual evoked response in diagnosis of multiple sclerosis. *British Medical Journal, 4,* 661–664.

Hecox, K., & Galambos, R. (1974). Brainstem auditory evoked responses in human infants and adults. *Archives of Otolaryngology, 99,* 30–33.

Jerger, J., Hayes, D., & Jordan, C. (1980). Clinical experience with auditory brainstem response and audiometry in pediatric assessment. *Ear and Hearing, 1,* 19–25.

Kornhuber, H.H., & Deecke, L. (1965). Hirn potentialanderungen bei Willkur-Bewegungen und passiven Bewegungen des Menschen: Bereitschafts potential und reafferente potentiale. [Brain potential changes with active and passive movement in man: Readiness potential and reafferent potential]. *Pflugers Archiv fuer Die Gesamte Physiologie des Menschen und der Tier, 284,* 1–17.

Kornhuber, H. and Deecke, L. (Eds.). (1980). *Progress in brain research* (Vol. 54), *Motivation, motor and sensory processes of the brain: Electrical potentials, behavior and clinical use.* New York: Elsevier.

McCallum, W.C., & Knott, J.R. (Eds.). (1976). *The responsive brain.* Bristol: Wright.

McCallum, W.C., & Knott, J.R. (Eds.). (1973). Event-related slow potentials of the brain: Their relations to behavior. *Electroencephalography and Clinical Neurophysiology,* Suppl. 33.

McFarland, R.A., Roughton, F.J.W., Halperin, M.H., & Niven, J.I. (1944). The effects of carbon monoxide and altitude on visual thresholds. *Journal of Aviation Medicine, 15,* 381–394.

Noel, P., & Desmedt, J. (1980). Cerebral and far-field somatosensory evoked potentials in neurological disorders involving the cervical spinal cord, brainstem, thalamus and cortex. In J. Desmedt (Ed.), *Clinical uses of cerebral, brainstem and spinal somatosensory evoked potentials. Progress in Clinical Neurophysiology, 7,* 205–230.

Otto, D.A. (Ed.). (1978). *Multidisciplinary perspectives in event-related brain potential research.* Publication No. EPA-600/9-77-043. Washington, DC: U.S. Government Printing Office.

Otto, D. (1983). The application of event-related slow brain potentials in occupational medicine. In R. Gilioli, et al. (Eds.), *Neurobehavioral methods in occupational health* (pp. 71–78). London: Pergamon Press.

Otto, D.A. (in press). The relationship of event-related brain potentials and lead absorption: A review of current evidence. In L. Wysocki and L. Goldwater (Eds.), *Lead environmental health: The current issues.*

Otto, D., Benignus, V., Muller, K., Barton, C. (1981). Effects of age and body lead burden on CNS function in young children. I. Slow cortical potentials. *Electroencephalography and Clinical Neurophysiology, 52,* 229–239.

Otto, D., Benignus, V., Muller, K., Barton, C., & Schroeder, S. (1982). Effects of low to moderate lead exposure on slow cortical potentials in young children. Two-year follow-up study. *Neurobehavioral Toxicology and Teratology, 4,* 733–737.

Otto, D., Benignus, V.A., & Prah, J.H. (1978). The paradoxical effects of carbon monoxide on vigilance performance and event-related potentials. In D. Otto (Ed.), *Multidisciplinary perspectives in event-related brain potential research* (pp. 440–443). Publication No. EPA-600/9-77-043, Washington, DC: U.S. Government Printing Office.

Otto, D., Benignus, V., Seiple, K., Loiselle, D., & Hatcher, T. (1980). ERPs in young children during sensory conditioning. In H. Kornhuber and L. Deecke (Eds.), *Motivation, motor and sensory processes of the brain: Electrical potentials, behavior and clinical use, Progress in Brain Research, 54,* 574–578.

Otto, D., & Reiter, L. (1978). Neurobehavioral assessment of environmental insult. In D. Otto (Ed.), *Multidisciplinary perspectives in event-related brain potential research* (pp. 409–416). Publication No. EPA-600/9-77-043. Washington, DC: U.S. Government Printing Office.

Otto, D., Robinson, G., Baumann, S., Schroeder, S., Mushak, P., Kleinbaum, D., & Boone, L. (1985). Five-year follow-up study of children with low-to-moderate lead absorption: Electrophysiological evaluation. *Environmental Research, 38,* 168–186.

Robinson, G., Baumann, S., Schroeder, S., Mushak, P., & Otto, D. (1985). Effects of low to moderate lead exposure on brainstem auditory evoked potentials in children. *Environmental Health,* Doc. 3, (pp. 177–182). Copenhagen: World Health Organization.

Schaumberg, H., Arezzo, J., Markowitz, L., and Spencer, P. (1981). Neurotoxicity assessment at chemical disposal sites. In W. Lowrance (Ed.), *Assessment of health effects at chemical disposal sites* (pp. 81–104). Los Altos, CA: W. Kaufmann.

Scherg, M., & Von Cramon, D. (1985). A new interpretation of the generators of BAEP waves I-V: Results of a spatio-temporal dipole model. *Electrocephalography and Clinical Neurophysiology, 62,* 290–299.

Schwartz, D.M., & Berry, G.A. (1985). Normative aspects of the ABR. In J.T. Jacobson (Ed.), *The auditory brainstem response* (pp. 65–97). San Diego: College-Hill Press.

Seppalainen, A.M. (1975). Applications of neurophysiological methods in occupational medicine: A review. *Scandinavian Journal of Work, Environment and Health, 1,* 1–14.

Seppalainen, A.M. (1978). Diagnostic utility of neuroelectric measures in environmental and occupational medicine. In D. Otto (Ed.), *Multidisciplinary perspectives in event-related brain potential research* (pp. 448–452). Washington, DC: U.S. Government Printing Office.

Seppalainen, A.M., Raitta, C., & Huuskonen, M.S. (1980). Nervous and visual effects of occupational n-hexane exposure. In H. Lechner and A. Aranibar (Eds.), *EEG and clinical neurophysiology* (pp. 656–661). Amsterdam: Excerpta Medica.

Sillman, A., Bolnick, D., Bosetti, J., Haynes, L., & Walter, A. (1982). The effects of lead and cadmium on the mass photoreceptor potential: The dose-response relationship. *Neurotoxicology, 3,* 179–194.

Sokol, S. (1976). Visually evoked potentials: Theory, techniques and clinical applications. *Surveys in Ophthalmology, 21,* 18–44.

Sokol, S. (1980). Visual evoked potentials. In M. Aminoff (Ed.), *Electrodiagnosis in clinical neurology* (pp. 348–369). New York: Churchill Livingston.

Sokol, S., & Jones, K. (1979). Implicit time of pattern evoked potentials in infants: An index of maturation of spatial vision. *Vision Research, 19*, 747–755.

Starr, A. (1977). Clinical relevance of brain stem auditory evoked potentials in brain stem disorders in man. *Progress in Clinical Neurophysiology, 2*, 45–57.

Starr, A., Sohmer, H., & Celesia, G.G. (1978). Some applications of evoked potentials to patients with neurological and sensory impairment. In E. Callaway, P. Tueting, & S. Koslow (Eds.), *Event-related brain potentials in man* (pp. 155–196). New York: Academic Press.

Sutton, S., Braren, M., & Zubin, J. (1965). Evoked potential correlates of stimulus uncertainty. *Science, 150*, 1187–1188.

Walter, W.G., Cooper, R., Aldridge, V.J., McCallum, W.C., & Winter, A.L. (1964). Contingent negative variation: An electric sign of sensorimotor association and expectancy in the human brain. *Nature, 203*, 380–384.

Wooten, B.R. (1972). Photopic and scotopic contributions to the human visually evoked cortical potential. *Vision Research, 12*, 1647–1660.

Biomedical Prevention of Mental Retardation

A Model State Plan

Robert Guthrie
and
Maureen Young

Mental retardation and developmental disabilities are present in each of us, although we usually think in such terms only of those more obviously disabled: the blind, epileptic, or those in wheelchairs. Thus, the mentally retarded are often arbitrarily defined as the two or three percent of the population with IQs below 70, especially by the professions—medical, educational, and legal. Yet, considering that there are hundreds of causes of mental retardation, environmental and genetic, it is very unlikely that any of us were not retarded to *some* degree in our mental development in early life. No doubt Albert Einstein could have considered most of the people he met to be retarded (a "relative" theory of mental retardation). This perspective is important in considering the effects of prevention programs.

Removal of an agent such as lead from the environment of young children can affect the early development of many thousands of children and the quality of their entire lives, if we are to accept the data from the recent national survey. Not only would we lower the incidence of more severe mental retardation, learning disorders, hyperactivity, and behavior problems, we would decrease the numbers of children who would have difficulty graduating from high school and entering university, professional, and graduate schools. The same broad range of effects should occur from education efforts aimed at pregnant women to decrease their alcohol consumption. Removal of alcohol from the fetal environment will prevent not only the obvious stigmata of fetal alcohol syndrome, but also the more subtle effects on development not seen at birth.

Fred Krause, former Executive Director of the President's Committee on Mental Retardation, has said: "The 1960s in the United States was the decade of federal legislation for programs for the mentally retarded; the 1970s was the decade of the rights movement that led to implementation of these programs; the 1980s will be the decade of prevention." We believe that he may be right about the 1980s, as the rapid expansion in the community of educational programs, intermediate care facilities, group homes, day treatment programs, and sheltered workshops, with the associated rapid rise in the costs of these programs in public funds, is increasing awareness of the need for primary prevention.

Primary prevention in infants and children of nonlethal, lifelong severely handicapping conditions is one of modern medicine's great challenges following the dramatic decrease in infant mortality already achieved during this century in industrialized countries. Not only is a chronic, severe handicap a tragedy for the individual and family affected, but a great burden is placed upon society. The cost of infant mortality is the loss of a productive life; the cost of a handicap—especially severe mental retardation—is much greater.

Over 10 years ago, the President's Committee on Mental Retardation stated that in the United States we should be able to prevent 50% of mental retardation by the end of this century through application of the knowledge we already possess.

Fifty years ago, the introduction of iodized salt was estimated to have reduced mental retardation in Switzerland by 20% through reduction of endemic cretinism. Use of iodized salt is so commonplace now that most of us have forgotten how dramatic this achievement was. Two decades later, specific prevention of an inherited form of mental retardation, phenylketonuria (PKU), by dietary control of phenylalanine blood levels was introduced by Bickel, Gerrard, and Hicksman (1953).

Among several thousand known inherited handicapping conditions in our species, several hundred have been characterized as *inborn errors of metabolism* and more are continuously being discovered. One of these is PKU. Detection in the newborn of certain of these rare metabolic abnormalities that cause preventable mental retardation and developmental disabilities began approximately 20 years ago with the introduction of a simple laboratory test for phenylketonuria by Guthrie (1961). PKU, inherited once in ten thousand births as an autosomal recessive condition, is an enzyme deficiency in the conversion of the essential amino acid phenylalanine to a second amino acid, tyrosine. Development of the fetus is normal, but after birth the evaluation of phenylalanine concentration in the blood and body fluid is associated with retardation of growth of intelligence. Early institution of dietary control of phenylalanine intake can result in prevention of this effect.

Acceptance of the test was attributable to several unique features:

a. Use of a dried blood spot on special filter paper permitted a punched out paper disc to replace a measured aliquot of blood for a quantitative test. Surprisingly, such a specimen had never been used in medicine before. This also permitted a single laboratory to receive specimens from an entire state or country for high volume screening. The specimen is used for simultaneous testing for a number of rare conditions.

b. By combining knowledge of microbial growth and molecular competition in intermediary metabolism, very simple, reliable, and quantitative *bacterial inhibition assays* were developed for PKU and several other conditions, each using a dried disc of blood.

c. Equipment developed for semiautomated use of the specimen further improved efficiency and reduced costs (Guthrie, 1972).

As a result, many millions of infants are being screened by many countries and thousands have been saved from mental retardation.

During the same period, the explosion of knowledge concerning human chromosome morphologic abnormalities and their relation to birth defects and developmental disabilities occurred, including the techniques for prenatal diagnosis by culturing cells from amniotic cells for chromosomal karyotyping. This permitted therapeutic abortion of the affected offspring.

For the past two decades, it has been possible to prevent most of the common contagious childhood diseases with potent, safe vaccines. Yet measles, rubella, and whooping cough are still occurring and causing major neurologic disease in various parts of the country because of apathy and ignorance on the part of the public—and some physicians—concerning the need for immunizations. Browder (1977) has described how programs in the state of Oregon have saved lives, prevented developmental damage to children, and saved Oregon taxpayers millions of dollars.

Rh hemolytic disease of the newborn infant has been completely preventable since Rh immune globin (RhIG) became available in 1968. If this is given to each Rh negative mother after each delivery of an Rh positive baby and after each abortion, she does not produce the Rh antibodies that can damage a subsequent Rh positve infant before it is born. The Centers for Disease Control (CDC) estimated that in 1974 7,000 children were born mentally retarded because of this disease. It has been estimated by MacCready (1977) that in 1977 only 80% of such mothers received this protection, and that in 1982 probably only 85% were protected (MacCready, 1982). MacCready (1977) also described the Connecticut Department of Health's monitoring program as producing a 99% RhIG utilization rate and a dramatic reduction in morbidity and mortality rates caused by this condition between 1969 and 1976.

An ancient and major cause of developmental damage before birth, the effect of alcohol consumed during pregnancy, has only recently been "discovered" in 1968 in France (Lemoiner, Harousseau, Borteryu, & Menuet, 1968) and in 1973 in the United States (Jones, 1977). In New York State, a Governor's Task Force estimated that 386 cases of fetal alcohol syndrome occurred annually, with an additional 1563 cases of fetal alcohol affected infants (Russell, 1980). Obviously, this condition is preventable, but only if education of the prospective mother is successful. In this undertaking, the role of the obstetrician is, of course, very important. Educational programs aimed at the public as well as the professions have been mounted in many parts of the country.

Another important development during this decade was the demonstration in the United Kingdom that the frequency of births of infants with severe neural tube defects could be sharply reduced through the new technique of maternal blood testing for alpha-fetoprotein. After pilot programs had first demonstrated the feasibility of this approach, a national program was mandated with governmental support. It has been estimated by Milunsky (1977) that approximately 75% of severe neural tube defects could be prevented in the U.S. (through prenatal diagnosis and therapeutic abortion) if a similar program were developed here. However, only a relatively few small programs have been carried out in our country because of the many differences between our country and Great Britain. This is very frustrating to all of us who would like to see the tragedy and suffering associated with neural tube defects reduced.

In contrast, significant progress has been made in the past decade in our country in programs concerning prenatal care, malnutrition in infants and children, protection of infants and children in automobiles, teenage education, and childhood lead poisoning.

Intensive care perinatal units have dramatically improved not only the survival rate of high risk, ill, and very small premature infants, but also the quality of life of these survivors. This improvement is attributable to the principles and concepts involved in regionalization of perinatal care, according to Gluck (1977).

Many publications concerning experimental animal studies have clearly demonstrated that severe undernutrition during pregnancy or early infancy produces permanent deficits in the development of the brain and central nervous system. It has been much more difficult to prove such effects in our own species, but much evidence indicates similar effects (Russo, 1977). Federally funded Special Supplemental Food Programs for Women, Infants, and Children (WIC) have been very effective in increasing the birthweight of infants born to high risk mothers (Susser, Stein, & Ruth, 1978).

For the past decade, it has been known that the leading cause of death in children under age 16 in our country, as well as a major cause of handicap, is accidents, and that the majority of accidents occur to children as passengers in cars. Severe head injury is especially likely to the infant and young child. Fortunately, half of our state legislatures have become active in trying to mandate use of suitable restraints and car seats, which have been demonstrated to prevent 90% of the damage, and at least nine states had passed laws at the time this was written.

Increasing attention has been given to health education of adolescent children in our schools including the information they need to avoid becoming parents of handicapped offspring. This is particularly necessary because of the simultaneous increase in consumption of cigarettes, alcohol, and other drugs, as well as the frequency of pregnancy among teenage students. The synergistic effect of these factors in causing an increase in the mentally retarded and developmentally disabled members of the next generation is obvious. A unique and impressive contribution to the education of this population is the educational program developed by Sara Litch (1978, 1979). This material has proven very effective in increasing the knowledge of prevention among hundreds of teachers and thousands of students in Indiana and has been adopted in several other states.

Other very recent developments in our knowledge of prevention are the discoveries of the most frequent form of mental retardation and, even more important, a method of preventing its occurrence. This is X-linked mental retardation, or the *fragile* X chromosome, so called because of the chromosome's appearance under a microscope. Turner and Turner (1974) and Sutherland (1977) revealed some of the reasons that there has always been a preponderance of males in severely retarded populations. Brown and associates (1982) also found that fragile X is one cause of autism. The same group found that this cause is apparently preventable because of the development of a technique by which fragile X can be demonstrated in cells obtained by amniocentesis (Jenkins et al., 1981).

The current decade has witnessed a very interesting phase concerning an old problem—that of childhood lead poisoning. We call this period the *rediscovery* of childhood lead poisoning. It is worth reviewing this problem at some length because it is so immense and yet so poorly understood by a majority of the public as well as the professional community.

Among the thousands of causes known and unknown of mental retardation and developmental disabilities, environmental agents are possibly more important than genetic. Among these, our attention is increasingly drawn to the many products of modern industry that pollute our environment. Lead is perhaps the oldest of these and still the most neglected. Lead comes from many sources, including leaded gasoline and old paint. The federal government estimates that 4%, or 1 in every 25 children under age 6 in the United States, has a dangerously high blood concentration of lead. Lead effects are subtle; usually no immediate symptoms are present, but recent strong evidence indicates that permanent deficits in intelligence and school achievement and increased behavior problems result. The government recommends annual screening of all preschool children, but only 3% are being tested at present. This manmade cause of developmental disability can be prevented by screening, prompt chelation treatment, and separating the child from the source of lead.

We have simplified a test using dried blood spots (Orfanos, Murphey, & Guthrie, 1977) developed by Piomelli and Davidow of Columbia University that detects both iron deficiency and lead poisoning by measuring a deficiency in hemoglobin synthesis, and are advocating its use by regional laboratories on specimens collected annually from all preschool children in a large region. This is similar to the approach we developed for newborn screening (Guthrie, 1980). Currently, we are researching a bacterial test for another red blood cell enzyme sensitive to lead for use with a second disc from the same blood spot to make the screening procedure more specific. Once the idea of collecting this type of specimen annually from every young child is accepted, this specimen will undoubtedly be used for other tests of health and environmental significance to permit prevention of other causes of developmental damage in children.

How much mental retardation (using the usual definition) can be prevented? The President's Committee on Mental Retardation (PCMR) stated in 1971 that 50% could be prevented by the end of this century. At a conference on prevention organized by the PCMR in 1977, Moser estimated that 29% of severe mental retardation could be prevented (1977). However, by adding fetal alcohol effect and X-linked mental retardation, the estimate would be approximately 40%.

What are the cost benefits of such prevention? With our current severe constraints on public health budgets, this is an important aspect. A French perinatal care program for the period 1970–1975 was estimated to have saved 8 francs for each franc invested (Lancet editorial, 1976).

The U.S. General Accounting Office has estimated that if the federal government invested $20 million annually in a countrywide regionalized newborn screening program (similar to that in Japan, for example), $400 million—or twenty times as much—would be saved annually in public funds used for care of those that would be affected without the program (Comptroller General, 1977).

Another indication came from the recent estimates by Provenzano (1980) of the total cost of care of those affected by lead exposure in the U.S.: on the order of one-half to one billion dollars per year. Of course, this is only for those we know are affected, when only 3% of children are being screened! Obviously, if we counted everyone that had been affected by lead, the cost would be many times greater. The largest amount spent so far by the government is approximately $10 million per year, only 1% of the above estimated cost of caring for the known victims.

For prevention of fetal alcohol effect, the New York State Governor's Task Force estimated that a reduction of incidence by one-third in New

York State would save the state $50 million per year. This was based on an annual estimate of 386 cases of the syndrome and three to four times more cases less severely affected (Russell, 1980).

For the State of Oregon, Browder (1977) described the rubella vaccine program that existed during the 1970–1973 epidemic. This epidemic without the immunization program would have affected 150 children with congenital rubella. The program cost $350,000. A conservative estimate for the various types of medical, educational, and life care services is $11,953,000, approximately 30 times the cost of the program. Browder estimated cost benefits for a national measles immunization program during a 10-year period at $130 million.

Thus, the cost benefits of prevention of these nonlethal handicapping conditions seem enormous, and would save taxpayers large sums if government agencies would invest even small amounts of funds compared with the rapidly increasing budgets devoted to care for the victims of these conditions. Instead of taking funds away from such service programs, this action would make more funds available for the smaller number needing services.

Because the case for prevention of developmental disabilities is compelling, several states have requested leadership and guidance from the President's Committee on Mental Retardation in developing comprehensive prevention programs. The PCMR believes that a model state plan for prevention based upon the research and experience described above can serve as a blueprint for individual states to use in drawing up effective and appropriate plans.

The diverse nature of the 50 states precludes the drafting of one prevention plan ideal for all. However, there are certain characteristics, processes, and programs intrinsic to a model state prevention plan. Inplementation of these elements within a particular state will—and should—reflect the unique resources and needs of that state.

Characteristics of a state that are relevant to a model plan include demographic and geographic features, political organization, epidemiologic data, economic conditions, availability and accessibility of research and service resources, strength of consumer organizations, and other factors such as involvement in federal, regional, or centralized prevention efforts.

MODEL STATE PLAN STRUCTURE

The Model Plan Work Group of the President's Committee on Mental Retardation's National Prevention Showcase and Forum (Atlanta, 1982) determined that, although there exist variations among the characteristics of states, one can identify those essential components of a model state plan for prevention that are consistent from state to state. These components include: establishment of a state commission for prevention—the keystone of the plan; gathering of state-specific demographic and epidemiological data related to the causes and incidence of mental retardation and comparison of these data to national figures; estimation of costs; development of funding mechanisms; integration of prevention into the existing service delivery system; coordination of prevention efforts at a high level of government; coordination of private and public sector prevention activities; and involvement of consumers at all phases of prevention planning and implementation.

These eight activities provide structural support for a state prevention action plan and set the stage for state-specific needs assessment and program development. With the planning structure firmly in place, selection of program goals and methods can begin.

Program design assumes knowledge of the ways to prevent mental retardation. *Crocker's Golden Twenty* (Crocker, 1982) categorizes the basic elements of a comprehensive prevention program under the headings of *primary, secondary,* and *tertiary prevention.* (Primary prevention aims to prevent a condition among the general population; secondary prevention focuses on a group known to be at risk for the condition; and tertiary prevention seeks to ameliorate the effects of that condition among those who have it.) The twenty elements that Crocker believes essential to a good prevention program are: primary—rubella immunization, prenatal care, special care of the premature, genetic counseling, advice about alcohol intake during pregnancy, reduction of exposure to lead, prevention of kernicterus, reduction of childhood accidents, reduction of teenage pregnancy, efforts to decrease child neglect and abuse, and health and nutrition education; secondary—screening of newborns for treatable metabolic problems, screening for hypothyroidism, amniocentesis for older mothers, screening for elevated alpha-fetaprotein level, and identification of carriers of genetic conditions related to retardation; tertiary—early intervention and stimulation, continuing provision of services to families of children with disabilities, continuing research regarding causes of retardation, and education of physicians and other professionals.

Crocker's Golden Twenty represent many different causes, target groups, and actions. By focusing on target groups and actions, the New York Governor's Conference for the Prevention of Developmental Disabilities and Infant Mortality has identified seven action arenas: public education and information; prevention services—maternal and infant health; services to populations with special needs; education for special groups; service coordination and integration; data and research for planning and evaluation; and implementation. For each of these topic areas, the New York Conference proposes a goal, one or more objectives and specific activities (New York Governor's Conference, 1981).

Prevention planning documents exist within other states. For example, Illinois has published *Prevention of Developmental Disabilities in Illinois: Options to Guide State Prevention Efforts* (Illinois Bureau of the Budget, 1979). Many of the elements of a comprehensive plan are included in state health departments' maternal and child health plans; other components can be found in state public aid or child welfare mandates.

The 11-Point Model State Plan that follows is a synthesis of Crocker's Golden Twenty, New York's Prevention Action Plan, Illinois' Options to Guide State Prevention Efforts, previous PCMR reports, and the recommendations of the PCMR Model State Plan Work Group.

MODEL STATE PLAN PROGRAMS

Allowing for regional differences in needs and resources and expecting (and indeed welcoming) diversity of program priorities and activities among the states, the President's Committee on Mental Retardation believes that each state plan should address 11 points in its program for prevention of mental retardation. These 11 points are public education, maternal and child preventive health services, nutrition programs, environmental protection, genetic services, newborn screening programs, developmental screening, coordination of prevention services, citizen advisory groups, research and evaluation, and legislation.

Public Education

Both the general public and specific groups within the public need basic information about the importance of medical care, nutrition, safety, and education for optimal child development. Groups requiring education oriented to their needs and societal roles include not only adolescents and parents, but also service providers, teachers, policy makers, government officials, legislators, and the media.

In other words, all persons responsible for the health and well being of children need both general and specific information about prevention of mental retardation. This information should include the *why, how,* and *what* of each specific prevention measure.

For example, in the area of child passenger safety, a public education campaign should alert adults and older children to the importance of car seats and seat belts, should demonstrate the proper use of such equipment, and should identify resources for locating the proper equipment (i.e., lending programs, thrift shops, consumer information groups, etc.). Similarly, in the area of immunizations, parents should understand that childhood diseases are dangerous, that shots can prevent many illnesses, and that shots are available through private physicians, clinics, or hospitals.

A comprehensive public education plan would address child health and safety and adolescent and adult reproductive health. As in any marketing campaign, the specific content and style of the education approach should be tailored to the unique needs of the target group. Thus, information on reproductive health would be presented differently to adolescents than to adults. Education of legislators about a pending newborn screening bill would take a different shape than education of hospital administrators or parents.

Public education stands as a separate program in a model state plan and as a factor in the implementation of each of the other 10 points. Informed consumers, policy makers, administrators, and caregivers are essential to the prevention of mental retardation.

Maternal and Child Preventive Health Services

"The provision of high quality prenatal, obstetrical, and neonatal care, and preventive services during the first year of life, can reduce a newborn's risk of illness and death. Of particular concern are adolescents, whose infants experience a high degree of low birth weight and whose health problems should be addressed in a broad context taking into consideration social and psychological considerations" (Public Health Service, 1980).

In *Promoting Health/Preventing Disease: Objectives for the Nation* (Public Health Service, 1980), 13 specific measures to improve the health status and reduce risk factors for women and young children were proposed. These included family planning, prenatal care, innovative multidisciplinary medical care systems, accessible services, regionalization of perinatal services, adequate linkages, outreach, evaluation of quality of perinatal and infant care, identification and tracking of infants and families with specific problems, reduction in teenage and other high risk pregnancies, elimination of unnecessary radiation exposure, adequate primary care, and support groups for parents of high risk infants and other parents under stress.

Another important facet of a maternal and child health service is primary care for children beyond the first year of life and through adolescence, including immunization and screening programs. Genetic and newborn screening programs, because of their specific relevance to prevention of mental retardation, are discussed separately within this document.

Nutrition Programs

"There is no finer investment for any community than putting milk into babies."—Winston Churchill

Participation in federally supported food programs, including WIC (Women, Infants, and Children), school lunch, and Head Start should be expanded. Nutrition education, along with the means for obtaining an appropriate diet, is also critical. Because nutritional status can combine with other causes of mental retardation, such as lead poisoning or phenylketonuria, to increase the risk of brain damage, it is essential that children who are at nutritional risk be identified and supplied with appropriate diets. Dietary supplements for children with inborn errors of metabolism, vitamins and calcium for pregnant and lactating women, and balanced diets for all children are but a few of the specific nutritional services a state can support.

Environmental Protection

The list of substances known to cause reproductive, neurologic, or other damages that can produce mental retardation is long and growing. Enforcement of existing environmental legislation, screening of women and children for undue absorption of toxic substances, and corrections of hazards where they are known to exist require a coordinated effort on the part of the administrative and regulatory agencies of the states and federal government. Specific actions that can reduce mental retardation include such practices as annual screening of all children ages 1 through 6 years for lead absorption, with appropriate follow-up medical and environmental corrections. Annual screening for blood lead levels should be included in any state plan for prevention.

Genetic Services

"Counseling of couples-at-risk before they have any children: counseling 'before the fact'; such should be a major goal of any genetic prevention program" (PCMR, 1980).

In its 1980 *Report to the President/Mental Retardation: Prevention Strategies That Work,* the PCMR (1980) identified five ways to prevent mental retardation caused by genetic factors: counseling for individuals at risk of having a retarded child, screening for metabolic disorders, screening of the normal population to identify carriers of genetic disorders, prenatal (fetal) diagnosis of genetic disorders, and early treatment of such disorders. Newborn screening and early treatment programs are discussed elsewhere in this document. Screening of the general population and testing, counseling, and follow-up services for persons at risk of having a mentally retarded child are often concentrated in large urban areas with university hospital resources. Expansion of existing programs and increased accessibility of genetic services should be addressed in a state prevention plan. If resources allow, the plan might also include support for genetic research.

Newborn Screening Programs

Richard Koch stated: "In California, there has not been a single PKU person admitted to our state institutions who was born after 1966, the year our screening program began" (Edwards, 1982).

Phenylketonuria, hypothyroidism, galactosemia, and other inborn errors of metabolism lead to mental retardation unless detected early in infancy and treated with appropriate diets. Centralized screening of all newborns has proven an effective prevention technique; where screening is done by a variety of laboratories, however, costs rise and efficiency decreases. In those areas of the country such as New England and the Northwestern states, which have formed regional metabolic screening programs, there have been not only an increase in efficiency and reduction in cost, but also an increase in the numbers of children and types of disorders screened for and consequent prevention of mental retardation.

Several states have established networks of and/or regional centers to advise parents and physicians on the dietary treatment and other supports necessary for children with metabolic disorders.

Each state plan should include a mechanism, whether internal or cooperative with other states or a combination thereof, for the screening, dietary supplements, medical care, and counseling necessary for children with metabolic disorders.

Developmental Screening

Medicaid eligible children are provided developmental screening through the federal Early and Periodic Screening, Diagnosis, and Treatment Program (EPSDT). EPSDT-type programs should be provided to all children within the state, regardless of income level, with children diagnosed as developmentally at risk, delayed, or disabled provided with appropriate early intervention programming.

Coordinated Services for Prevention

The services described above cut across traditional socioeconomic and political boundaries. The state agency with responsibility for coordination of the overall prevention plan must design service plans and allocate resources in order to ensure accessibility for all state residents. In some states, a prevention circuit may be designed with interdisciplinary teams providing services on a frequent schedule in rural communities. Other states may arrange a transportation system. The unique characteristics of the state and experience with other statewide programs can suggest the solutions to accessibility problems.

Advisory Group on Implementation of Prevention Programs

To ensure that the state's prevention programs are meeting the needs of the population and that designated state agencies are cooperating with each other and with consumers and private sector service providers, a state advisory group for prevention should be established. This group should be composed of individuals and agency representatives reflective of the demographics and resources of the particular state. The advisory group should be charged with a watchdog function to ensure interprogram communication and coordination of services and to address specific problems as they arise. This advisory group might be a part of a commission on prevention or it might be a separate entity with representation on the commission.

Research and Evaluation

A specific state program, office, or agency should be given the responsibility and held accountable for coordinating prevention research and evaluation within the state. Each state should: gather and disseminate demographic and epidemiologic data about mental retardation, philosophically and financially support basic research programs in fetal development, undertake applied research on effectiveness of specific prevention strategies, and study the cost/benefit ratio of the various prevention initiatives. Some states may find that these efforts can best be handled through a regional research program supported by two or more neighboring states. In every instance, however, specific state agencies or subcontractors responsible for a component of the overall prevention plan of the state must provide for an evaluation component for their specific area(s) of responsibility.

Finally, the research and evaluation office should communicate program results and new knowledge to appropriate agencies, individuals, and the general public in a timely and suitable fashion. The new information developed through experience and research will strengthen the foundations of both the public education program and the public education initiatives of all the varied components of a model state plan for prevention.

Legislation

Prevention of disabilities can often be addressed most effectively through legislation or regulation. Mandatory immunization of children, use of child passenger restraints, removal of lead from household paint, newborn screening, and other prevention measures have, in many states, contibuted to a decrease in certain types of mental retardation. Each state should develop a mechanism for the consideration of prevention legislation as part of the ordinary business of the state.

Prevention is not a single issue, but a complex blend of medical, social, educational, and economic concerns. Prevention must join highways, schools, and natural resources as a perennial legislative concern. A state with a demonstrated commitment to the prevention of disabilities can take pride in its values and accomplishments.

PRIORITIES

A comprehensive state plan for prevention will necessitate choices. The Western New York Task Force on Prevention of Developmental Disabilities has developed seven criteria for prevention action (Edwards, 1985) to assist in prevention program development. These criteria are:

a. *The cause of the developmental disability and the means of prevention are well understood*. For example, injuries from car crashes are a leading cause of brain damage and the use of child passenger safety restraints can frequently prevent injury.

b. *A significant number of cases is produced*. In the preceding example of injuries from car crashes, the number of cases is overwhelmingly significant, as car crashes are a leading cause of death and serious injury for children. In other instances, such as phenylketonuria, which affects approximately 1 in 15,000 babies, the number becomes significant when considered in the light of human and economic costs: lifetime care of one child with PKU will cost a state an estimated $1,000,000. Thus, one case is a significant number.

c. *The cost is reasonable.* Some prevention methods, such as newborn screening, lead screening, and immunizations, are relatively inexpensive. For some families, however, $40 to $50 for a child passenger safety seat may seem like an unreasonable sum of money. When balanced against the risk of injury and the cost of medical and supportive care for an injured child, however, the cost can be justified. Reasonableness of cost should be approached from a broad perspective and with a view toward long term costs of failure to prevent a specific condition.

d. *Cooperation of the public and professionals is likely; little controversy is expected.* Lest the many noncontroversial prevention activities described here and elsewhere become lost in the chasm between polarized groups, state prevention programs should exercise caution before embarking on controversial projects. Value judgments will be made in any prevention program; these judgments, however, should reflect a sensitivity to the democratic and pluralistic society for which the state exists.

e. *A definite gap in services exists.* Some states have no newborn screening program, others have comprehensive programs, and some fall in-between. A state that screens for 12 metabolic disorders may turn to issues such as genetic research, whereas a state with little or no screening program may assign this a top priority.

f. *Model programs exist.* Although some states will want to develop model programs and are encouraged to do so, a newly formed state prevention program should begin with proven models. For the prevention initiative to survive and flourish, early success is crucial. Furthermore, replication or adaptation of a successful model is generally less expensive than the development of a new model.

g. *It will be possible to measure success.* In a comprehensive state plan for prevention, many components must coalesce and function effectively. Success can be measured in terms of both the structure and the effectiveness of the plan and its objectives. For example, structural success may include the formation of a legislative commission for prevention or the signing of an interagency or interstate cooperative agreement. Effectiveness of prevention programs can be measured in the short term for such activities as newborn screening (the annual number of PKU children identified early and treated effectively) or the long term (the incidence of mental retardation among the children of parents who received target prevention education as adolescents, compared with the general population).

SUMMARY

A model state plan for prevention coordinates human, economic, and social resources in a thoughtful process of identification of causes and prevention of mental retardation and a systematic application of that knowledge through a variety of approaches.

> Systems approaches suggest that "everything is connected to everything else." In this connection, a program, by definition, should be a planned effort to approach various aspects of an identified major problem by means of a series of interrelated projects; a single, isolated, one-shot project is not a program. This definition of program connotes a sustained commitment consistent with planned social change in order to modify institutions to make them more responsive to community need (Goldston, 1977).

A *sustained commitment* is the cornerstone of a model state plan for prevention. The meshing of effort and services demanded of comprehensive prevention planning requires the support of both the executive and legislative branches of government.

REFERENCES

Bickel, H., Gerrard, J., & Hicksman, E.M. (1953). Influence of phenylalanine intake on phenylketonuria. *Lancet, II*, 313.

Browder, J.A. (1977). Immunizations and what can be done to improve their use. *Proceedings of an International Summit on Prevention of Mental Retardation from Biomedical Causes* (pp. 153–161). Racine, Wisconsin. Washington, DC: Department of Health, Education, and Welfare [HEW Publication No. (HDS) 78-21023].

Brown, W.T., Jenkins, E.C., Friedman, E., Brooks, J., Wisniewski, K., Raguthu, S., & Frence, J. (1982). Autism is associated with fragile-X syndrome. *Journal of Autism and Developmental Disorders, 12*, 303–308.

California Association for the Retarded. (1977). *Prevention: An agenda for action* (p. 59). Sacramento, CA: Author.

Churchill, Winston. Radio broadcast, March 21, 1943. In *Oxford Dictionary of Quotations* (2nd ed.), p. 144, line 14. London: Oxford University Press.

Crocker, A.C. (1982). Current strategies in prevention of mental retardation. *Pediatric Annals, 11*, 450–457.

Editorial. (1976). French lessons on handicap. *Lancet, II*, 941.

Edwards, J. (1985). Community education project: Prevention of mental retardation and developmental disabilities. In J.H. Koch (Ed.), *Technical proceedings: President's National Showcase and Forum*. Washington, DC: Department of Health and Human Services.

Goldston, S.E. (1977). An overview of primary prevention programming. In D.C. Klein & S.E. Goldston (Eds.), *Primary prevention: An idea whose time has come* (pp. 23–40). Washington, DC: HEW Public Health Service.

Gluck, P. (1977). Regionalization of perinatal care. *Proceedings of an International Summit on Prevention of Mental Retardation from Biomedical Causes* (pp. 136–143). Racine, Wisconsin. Washington, DC: Department of Health, Education, and Welfare [HEW Publication No. (HDS) 78-21023].

Guthrie, R. (1961). Blood screening for phenylketonuria. *Journal of the American Medical Association, 178,* 863.
Guthrie, R. (1972). Mass screening for genetic disease. *Hospital Practice, 7,* 93–100.
Guthrie, R. (1980). Organization of a regional newborn screening laboratory. In H. Bickel, R. Guthrie, & G. Hammersen (Eds.), *Neonatal screening for inborn errors of metabolism* (pp. 259–270). Heidelberg: Springer-Verlag.
Illinois Bureau of the Budget. (1979). *Prevention of developmental disabilities in Illinois: Options to guide state prevention efforts.* Springfield, IL: Office of Planning.
Jenkins, E.C., Brown, W.T., Duncan, C., Brooks, J., Ben-Yishay, M., Giordano, F.N., & Nitowsky, H.M. (1981). Feasibility of fragile-X chromosome prenatal diagnosis demonstrated. *Lancet, II,* 1292.
Jones, K.L. (1977). Maternal alcoholism and fetal abnormalities. *Proceedings of an International Summit on Prevention of Mental Retardation from Biomedical Causes* (pp. 169–176). Racine, Wisconsin. Washington, DC: Department of Health, Education, and Welfare [HEW Publication No. (HDS) 78-21023].
Lemoine, P., Harousseau, H., Borteryu, J.P., & Menuet, J.C. (1968). Les enfants des parents alcooliques. Anomalies observees apropos des 127 cas. *Quest Medical, 25,* 476.
Litch, S. (1978). *Towards the prevention of mental retardation in the next generation,* Vol. I. Fort Wayne, IN: East Allen County Schools.
Litch, S. (1979). *Towards the prevention of mental retardation in the next generation,* Vol. II. Fort Wayne, IN: East Allen County Schools.
MacCready, R.A. (1977). Prevention of Rh hemolytic disease. *Proceedings of an International Summit on Prevention of Mental Retardation from Biomedical Causes* (pp. 78–81). Racine, Wisconsin. Washington, DC: Department of Health, Education, and Welfare [HEW Publication No. (HDS) 78-21023].
MacCready, R.A. (1982). Private communication.
Milunsky, A. (1977). A national program to prevent neural tube disorders. *Proceedings of an International Summit on Prevention of Mental Retardation from Biomedical Causes* (pp. 27–36). Racine, Wisconsin. Washington, DC: Department of Health, Education, and Welfare [HEW Publication No. (HDS) 78–21023].
Moser, H. (1977). Prevention of mental retardation from biomedical causes. *Proceedings of an International Summit on Prevention of Mental Retardation from Biomedical Causes* (pp. 2–5). Racine, Wisconsin. Washington DC: Department of Health, Education, and Welfare.
New York State Governor's Conference for the Prevention of Developmental Disabilities and Infant Mortality. (1981). *Prevention action plan* (pp. 79–102). Albany, New York. State of New York Publication.
Orfanos, A.P., Murphey, W.H., & Guthrie, R. (1977). A simple fluorometric assay of protoporphyrin in erythrocytes (EPP) as a screening test for lead poisoning. *Journal of Laboratory and Clinical Medicine, 89,* 659–665.
President's Committee on Mental Retardation. (1980). *Report to the President/Mental retardation: Prevention strategies that work* (p. 59). Washington, DC: Department of Health and Human Services [Publication No. DHHS(OHDS) 80–21029].
Provenzano, G. (1980). The social costs of excessive lead exposure during childhood. In H.L. Needleman (Ed.), *Low level lead exposure: The clinical implications of current research* (pp. 299–315). New York: Raven Press.
Public Health Service. (1980). *Promoting health/Preventing disease: Objectives of the nation* (p. 15). Washington, DC: Department of Health and Human Services Publication.
Report to the Congress by the Comptroller General of the United States. (1977). *Prevention of mental retardation—More can be done* [Report HRD-77–37, October 3, 1977]. Washington, DC: United States General Accounting Office.
Rosso, P. (1977). Nutrition, brain growth, and prevention of mental retardation. *Proceedings of an International Summit on Prevention of Mental Retardation from Biomedical Causes* (pp. 89–100). Racine, Wisconsin. Washington, DC: Department of Health, Education, and Welfare [HEW Publication No. (HDS) 78–21023].
Russell, M. (1980). Impact of alcohol-related birth defects (ARBD) on New York State. *Neurobehavioral Toxicology, 2,* 277–283.
Susser, M., Stein, Z.A., & Ruth, D. (1978). Prenatal nutrition and subsequent development.

In P. Mittler & J.M. deJong (Eds.), *Research to practice in mental retardation: Proceedings of the Fourth Congress of the International Association for the Scientific Study of Mental Deficiency: Vol. 3. Biomedical aspects*. Baltimore, MD: University Park Press.

Sutherland, G.P. (1977). Fragile sites of human chromosomes: Demonstration of their dependence on the type of tissue culture medium. *Science, 197*, 265–266.

Turner, G., & Turner, B. (1974). X-linked mental retardation. *Journal of Medical Genetics, 11*, 109–113.